STEM CELLS
THE HEALING REVOLUTION

Chronic Pain Relief and Regeneration without Drugs or Surgery

Discover how to eliminate knee,
hip, shoulder, and other chronic pain.

DR. RAJ BANERJEE

Published by Raj Banerjee

St. Louis, MO USA

Printed in United States of America

ISBN 979-1-949535-0909

This publication is designed to provide accurate and authoritative information with regard to the subject matter covered. It is sold with the understanding that the publisher is not engaged in rendering legal, accounting, or other professional advice. If legal advice or other expert assistance is required, the services of a competent professional should be sought.

For more information call Regenerative Health Medicine of St. Louis LLC at (314) 282-3990

Visit us online at: www.RegenHealthMed.com

DISCLAMER

THIS BOOK IS INTENDED FOR INFORMATIONAL PURPOSES ONLY.

Tissue therapy and biological cellular therapy is what most people think of when people hear the term stem cell therapy. Even though stem cell therapy is not the full description of tissue therapy and biological cellular therapy, it is what most people know and recognize, so we will be using the term "STEM CELLS" throughout this book to reference tissue therapy and biological cellular therapy.

We are not charactering regenerative medicine as just stem cells as that would be inaccurate. The labs we partner with continues to research and analyze the intricate relationship of contributing factors needed to help the body repair, replace, cushion, support, protect and function at optimal levels. It's that thorough understanding of all the parts that make the whole that enables us to recommend market leading products.

The body's regenerative process requires a dynamic environment consisting of a variety of growth factors, cytokines, scaffolding, hyaluronic acids, mesenchymal stem cells and chemokines. So in the event of injury, the body relies upon more than just a stem cell. It needs the complex rally of many cells and proteins to help start or aid the regenerative process and get it back up to speed. That's where we come in, replenishing what the body needs, where the body needs it, to better maintain the whole.

Stem cell therapy is not a cure or treatment for any disease or condition. Stem cells are a natural resource in the human body and they deplete over time. Professional judgment and expertise is needed in using stem cells for any therapeutic use, and we urge anyone embarking on the use of stem cell therapies to consult the national health data bases to evaluate current information from clinical trials, and the FDA websites on human tissue should also be consulted to get its current evaluation of any therapy.

In accordance with the FTC guidelines concerning the use of endorsements and testimonials in advertising, please be aware of the following. Federal regulations require us to advise you that all reviews, testimonials, and/or endorsements of any kind reflect the personal experience of those individuals who have expressed their own personal opinions, and those opinions and experiences may not be representative of what every consumer may personally experience with the endorsement. All reviews and testimonials are the sole opinions, findings, and/or experiences of the people sharing their stories. The people are not compensated in any way. These statements have not been evaluated by the US Food and Drug Administration (FDA). We are required to inform you that there is no intention—implied or otherwise—that represents or infers that these statements be used in the cure, diagnosis, mitigation, treatment, and/or prevention of any disease. These success stories do not imply that similar results would or could happen for you. These success stories are not intended to diagnose for specific illnesses or conditions or be a treatment to eliminate diseases or other medical conditions or complications. Names and details of their stories have been changed to protect their privacy, and any similarity between the names and stories of individuals described in this book and individuals known to readers is purely coincidental.

The statements in this book about consumable products or food have not been evaluated by Food and Drug Administration or other regulatory agencies. The publisher is not responsible for your specific health or allergy needs that may require medical supervision. The publisher is not responsible for any adverse reactions to the consumption of food or products that have been suggested in the book.

We make no medical claims as to the benefits of anything to improve medical conditions. Neither the author nor the publisher are engaged in rendering professional advice to the individual reader. The information in this book should not be regarded as a substitute for professional medical treatment. As with any medical treatment, results will vary among individuals, and there is no implication that you will heal, improve, run a marathon, play professional sports, or receive the same outcome as patients herein. Although very unlikely, there could be risks involved. These concerns should be discussed with your health care provider prior to any treatments so that you have proper informed consent and understand that there are no guarantees to healing. Neither the author nor the publisher shall be liable or responsible for any loss or damage allegedly arising from any information or suggestion in this book

This book is dedicated to my mom and to my dad. They have been my biggest source of encouragement as they have taught me that the greatest purpose in life is to serve and help others.

I also dedicate this book to all my wonderful former patients, and to all those who are truly ready to transform their lives.

And lastly, I dedicate this book to God, for I wouldn't have been able to complete this book without divine support and inspiration that is channeled through all that welcome and honor God's gracious gifts and Insights.

For more information on becoming a patient
or starting the Stem Cell Enhancement Program
please visit:

www.RegenHealthMed.com/StartHere

or Call:
314-282-3990

For more information on the newest stem
cell supplement called StemVantage please visit:

www.NutriHealthLabs.com

Use discount code

"save30"

to save $30 on your first
purchase of StemVantage.

Real Patients. Real Results -
The Healing Revolution

"My Whole Body Feels Better After One Injection..."

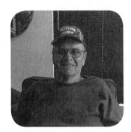

"I had Stem Cell therapy for my hip pain six weeks ago and it's performed magnificently!

I had one injection and helped my other hip and my other joints are feeling better, my shoulders, my hands and ankles. I have rheumatoid arthritis and matter of fact my whole body feels better from one injection."

~ Ted

"Before I Couldn't Walk,
Now I feel 10 YEARS Younger
After One Treatment..."

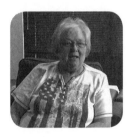

"I came to see Dr. Banerjee because I couldn't walk anymore. I was not able to walk anymore because my right knee was hurting so bad. I got the stem cell injection and that very evening, I immediately felt a difference. It's been AWESOME! I walked around for 4 hours to the zoo with my grandchildren. Which I would never have been able to do.

In the last 6 weeks my kidney function has improved and my overall body inflammation, which is monitored by a blood test from my doctor, has improved. So I am just really thrilled by my results. And I have pulmonary hypertension which leads to shortness of breath and I am not having shortness of breath anymore.

I feel younger! I feel 10 YEARS younger than I did 6 weeks ago. I recommend it highly!

~ Sandra

"I Don't Wake Up With Pain Anymore! I Can Sleep All Night Now!"

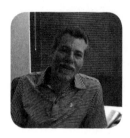

"I have had shoulder pain for over twenty years and absolutely nothing helped. When I heard about Dr. Raj Banerjee's stem cell therapy I jumped on and I am glad I did.

I have diabetes, I have shoulder pain, I have hip pain, and I started getting arthritis in my hands. After two injections and few weeks later, I don't wake up in pain anymore. It's remarkable!

I sleep all night now. I don't wake up with pain in the morning. So that's a big bonus for me right there, is feeling rested waking up. And I can go about my daily activates without any pain in my shoulders.

My toes were turning purple on the ends because of my diabetes. I have been using insulin for 10 years now. And within two days, the purple color was gone. My toes got back to their natural color. They are not sensitive to pain anymore.

I just can't say enough about the stem cell therapy and how much it helped me out.

~ Ron

"I Could Hardly Walk... My Orthopedic Doctors Said I Needed Four Surgeries."

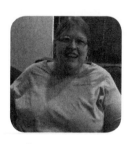

"Before I came here I could hardly walk. I had pain everywhere. I had two really bad knees and had Bonne on bone on my ankle, also feet pain. My orthopedic doctors were telling me that I needed four surgeries.

I am really glad I found Dr. Banerjee and his stem cell therapy. I was looking at four surgeries in my future. After two injections the pain is gone . My foot was the worst because they were bone on bone, and they were going to do surgery right away with that. And I said 'I got to do something different'.

So I came here and tried stem cells and I now walk. I used to walk with a cane all the time and now I can walk without needing a cane. It doesn't hurt at all anymore.

My whole body feels better. I think the stem cells are traveling throughout my body. I felt I was crippled whenever I got off work. I feel so much better now. I am so glad I did this."

~ Nancy

"I've Had Multiple Nerve Surgeries and Nothing Worked Until I Tried Stem Cells..."

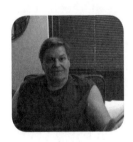

"I Have been having lot of knee pain and nerve pain, and came to try the stem cells. Was very skeptical, didn't think they would work. After doing them, I had them done in my knee and my nerve area, where I've had nerve pain, and the pain is down to nothing now. Nerve pain is gone. Knee pain is gone, so everything seems to be working.

I had a compound fracture, so I have a titanium rod in my leg. I've had multiple nerve surgeries and none of them really worked. We really didn't think this would work, but it was something to try. We tried it and it worked.

I was very skeptical. I didn't believe any of it when I came to a seminar. I said, "This isn't going to work." After a little bit of thinking about it, and people saying, "Well what do you got to lose?" I decided to give it a try.

I'm really glad I done it. Everybody I've talked to is really impressed with how it's been working. I used to be wake up at night with pain, with severe nerve pain, and knee pain. That's all gone now. I can sleep now. My wife is happy about that.

I very happy about the results. If I'm a non-believer and it turned me around, what would happen with a believer?"

~ Mike

"I'm 96% Better. I Love It! The Pain is Almost All Gone..."

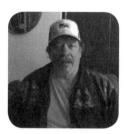

"I went to Dr. Banerjee back before Valentine's Day, and I got my shots on Valentine's Day. I'm like 96% better. I love it. The pain is almost all gone. It isn't like the kick in the shorts when you're just standing there and your back spasms, and you want to go to your knees. It's been great. I love it. I'd recommend this to anybody. It's been six weeks since the shots and it is just great.

My vision is a lot better. I got the IV push and after that I went home. We was relaxing and I was talking to the wife. I go, "Colors are so much better. They're more brighter." Not that my vision is perfect, but it was, oh the color came back. It was great. I love going out in the woods now because you can see the colors and everything. In this time of year it's great.

~ Mark

"You Don't Realize How Much Pain You Are In Until It's All Gone..."

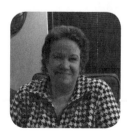

"I cannot believe how much pain I was in that I didn't even realize how bad it was until it was gone. Just going to a store, going to the grocery store, or a Walmart, or whatever, I would have to plan my trips where I could get in and out and only what I needed. And I would come out in severe pain limping. Then I would be home, get off my feet, feet in the air, miserable for the rest of the night.

I also work in sales, so there are days I'm on my feet all day, and I'm up and down steps. The look on my face when I would get home, people would say, "What's the matter?" It was just the amount of pain I was in. I'd be limping around for several days until the inflammation went down. I don't really have that. It doesn't do that anymore. I'm exercising now. Eating better, and it is making such a difference in my life. It is continuously getting better.

I would absolutely recommend Dr. Banerjee's program for others. I wish I could have got more. If I can, I will. This was so worth it.

~ Karen

"I Had Severe Hip Pain and Was Right on the Cusp of Having to Get Hip Replacement Surgery..."

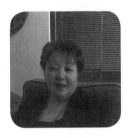

I'm Judy. I'm 61-years-old. I saw Dr. Banerjee on Facebook on an ad, and being very interested in it, and decided to go to a seminar, take my husband along. We went and was really intrigued, a little bit skeptical, but intrigued, and decided to go ahead and get the book which I read from cover to cover. And made an appointment.

We came in and I had been in a lot of pain in my left hip for probably six or seven years, and I was right on the cusp of having to get replacement surgery. I didn't want to do that. I had had open heart surgery about four years ago. I did not want to have any kind of surgery again after that. I was pretty much willing to do, to try anything.

After reading the book, I was very intrigued by the science that was involved. We decided to go ahead. I had not been able to walk around the block. Going downstairs was very difficult. I had almost gotten to the point where my pain level was between seven and eight 100% of the time. Like I say, I'm only 61-years-old, I have very young grandchildren and this was not going to be acceptable.

I had just one injection in my left hip. I didn't feel really too much relief immediately. It was probably 3 weeks before I started noticing going up and down stairs was not so much of a problem. I came in for my next appointment, and was told to go ahead and follow some of the other instructions that he gave me.

Now, it's been 12 weeks and I have absolutely NO PAIN!

In fact, I was making dinner with my kids, which is very hard for me to do, stand up for long periods of time. I actually got through making dinner and I had to just stop because I was in no pain. That never happens. I was able to go to the Flying Spider, which is this trampoline place with my grandkids, and then we went swimming, carrying my kids. It's like I've been given a new lease, life, living, just doing normal things that I thought was pretty much out of the question for me without having to go through surgery.

I would recommend this. Do the research. Read the book. The book is very eye opening. Listen to his seminars, listen to his videos. Get as much information as you need, because I'm telling you, this is really a life changing event for me.

~ Judy

"My Ankle Was Bone on Bone. After One Stem Cell Injection, No Pain and I'm Walking Normal Now..."

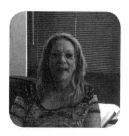

"Hi, my name's Jo Ellen and I've had the stem cell like six weeks ago. I've had a lot of trouble with my foot and my ankle is bone on bone. I have tremors and trouble breathing. I also have problems with my vocal cords. I have noticed that the stem cell therapy helped my ankle tremendously. I don't have the pain shooting down my knee, or the pain shooting from my foot down into my toe. My breathing has gotten better. I don't have rapid heartbeat anymore.

I have had a lot of extreme pain in my foot where I was limping all the time. That's one thing that I've noticed is that I've started walking like from heel to toe without having all this pain. I'm actually walking normal. That's the huge benefit that I've seen so far.

~Jo Ellen

"My Arthritis Was Getting So Bad, and the Amount of Meds I Was Taking, I Felt Like My 90 Year Old Dad..."

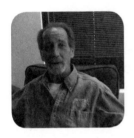

I'm Jim. I'm 59. I've been an electrician for 39 years. I do a lot on my knees, bending down, a lot of work with my hands. I've had such terrible arthritis in the past couple years, especially my hands, my knees and my ankles. After reading Dr. Banerjee's book, it really hit home. It really made me interested in finding that this is probably what's going to work for me.

I've been on medications, which gives me terrible side effects. The medications was just not working. That's why I decided to go for the stem cells. After having it done, it's been six weeks, I've noticed a great improvement in my hands to where they're not so stiff. I do a lot of tedious stuff with data work, and putting outlets on, and wiring, and they are not so stiff anymore.

My knee is where I had the injection and I haven't had any problems with that. I had gout in my feet and that's also getting better.

I only had one injection, one in my knee, and then one intravenously. I wanted to flood my body with stem cells because I have arthritis everywhere, my feet, my ankles, my hands, my neck, my shoulders. And I wanted to avoid any type of surgeries. My arthritis was getting so bad and the amount of medication I was taking made me feel like my dad, who is 90-years-old.

The meds gave me terrible diarrhea. I would be ready to go to work, and then I would have a spout, and I had to go back and change clothes. That's totally been gone since I quit taking the anti-inflammatory drugs. I haven't had any issues with that. I quit taking all my pain killers because I don't need it anymore.

I would recommend the book to read first because the more knowledge you have on anything, the better. Then you can make the decision whether to go for it or not.

I would definitely recommend Dr. Banerjee's stem cell program. Like I said, I'm for it, it really did well for me.

~ Jim

"I Don't Have Arthritis Pain Anymore. I'm Running With My Grandsons. I'm a New Person..."

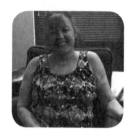

I have suffered from osteoarthritis, I would say probably at least 35, maybe 40 years of my life. It's genetic. It runs in the family. I also have done things in my past, I was a marathon runner. I ran on concrete and sidewalk, and you're not supposed to do that. Time marches on and I'm now 64. The arthritis has gotten worse, much worse.

I've had a knee replacement in the right knee, and a partial knee replacement in my left knee. I've also had a hip replacement on my left side. I had this opportunity, I'm leaving on a trip to Europe, on my bucket list. I wanted to be able to walk. I'm not going to miss a thing. I'm not going to sit in the hotel and, "Oh, my knees hurt too bad." I started doing research. I went to a lot of doctors. So many doctors were immediately suggested surgery, another knee replacement.

I just didn't want to go that route. I had some friends start talking about stem cell shots. I have a girlfriend that had one done. She had trouble with her knee. I was so impressed by how she was walking. I did a lot of research. This is how I found Dr. Banerjee. He seemed the most impressive. He seemed the most knowledgeable.

I thought, what do I have to lose? I could finance it. I came in and in prep for my trip, I had a stem cell shot in my left knee. This is the one that has the partial. I just cannot believe how wonderful it's been. It's the best thing I've ever done. I am more active. I don't have the headaches I used to have. I don't have the low back pain, which comes with old age and arthritis. That has subsided 60-70%. I have my energy back. I'm very active now. If I don't work out at the gym, I take at least a five mile walk every day.

I honestly don't think that I would be able to be where I'm at today if I hadn't had the stem cell shot. I would recommend it to anyone. The financing is very reasonable. It's not in the trillions. You can afford it and you would be very, very glad that you did.

Dr. Banerjee is also a fountain of knowledge. He knows arthritis. He knows pain. I'm still pondering possibly getting a stem cell shot in my right knee when I get back.

I would say right here and now, I leave in 10 days, I'm ready to go. I've never been out of the country. I think my walking is going to be terrific. I feel 100% better. I would suggest it to anybody. I have lost 10 pounds in five weeks.

I don't have arthritis pain. I don't have pain. Isn't that the idea to live life, and live life comfortably? I'm a new person. People have pointed it out to me like close friends, and my son. And now I'm running with my grandsons. That's probably a first of many things that have improved. It has changed my life. It's changed my life totally. So many things have improved. Just my whole level of pain, and then that affects your mood. It affects how you feel. When you don't have pain you want to get up in the morning. You want to do things.

~ Jeannie

"The Pain and Swelling is All Gone..."

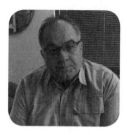 I am a disabled veteran. I returned from the Iraq War in 2005 with a number of illnesses. Some of those were fibromyalgia and arthritis. It got to the point within the last few years that my mobility was severely decreased. On some days it was all I could do to walk around in my own home. Around February 14th, I underwent the stem cell replacement therapy here with Dr. Banerjee.

Since then, my mobility has greatly increased; my pain level has gone down to almost non-existent. If it wasn't for this treatment, my only other recourse, because I had tried so many other therapies, medicines, treatments that didn't work, or didn't last for any length of time, was to move to a drier desert like climate, which I was all prepared to do. Since then, and this therapy, I now can remain here in the Midwest and live out my life here with my family.

My greatest pain was in my hands was where I had the most severe arthritis, but also the levels in my lower back, and in my knees, and feet were such that on some days the pain level was anywhere from a seven to a nine or ten. That greatly decreased my mobility. The pain levels are now less than one.

I received the one injection, which was put in my lower back. That had other effects elsewhere as in my hands. I had swelling throughout my body, including my feet. My hands felt the worse though. The pain and swelling is all gone.

I most certainly would recommend this for other people. If you're a veteran and you're in a lot of joint pain, this works.

~ Jack L.

"I Was Very Skeptical.
I Didn't Expect My Shoulder Pain
to Go Away So Quickly..."

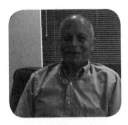 This is my sixth week checkup. And my shoulder pain is gone. We're talking about a rotator cuff in my shoulder. The movement I'm doing right now, I was not able to do. I hope whoever is seeing this will understand I'm not trying to exaggerate, but the injury was decades old.

When I was younger, I would put my arm under my pillow, over my head when I would sleep. That was just a comfortable way for me to sleep. For decades, I couldn't do this. It would wake me up at night, the pain would wake me up at night. I would do the wrong thing and it would wake me up. Then I would have the pain for a while, and take forever to go back to sleep.

After one injection my pain was gone very quickly. I guess the stem cells deal with the pain right away. I don't know. I can say this, it fooled me because I didn't know what to expect, and I was probably very skeptical. I didn't expect to have that kind of a change so quickly. As far as I'm concerned, this method of treating injury is amazing. I was a skeptical person. I did a lot of research, besides reading Dr. Banerjee's book.. I felt it was something I needed to try, as opposed to going through surgery, and then physical therapy to break the joint loose after they fix it.

I'm very happy. I have recommended this to a lot of folks. I think one very important thing is to follow all of the instructions after the injection. I did go off of a lot of supplements that were anti-inflammatory in nature. They were natural supplements, because I didn't want to confuse the stem cells. I think that's really important to follow the direction that Dr. Banerjee gives. I'm very happy with what's happened, and I'm going to recommend it to a lot of friends.

~ Glenn

"I Am a Nurse. I Know How Rheumatoid Arthritis is Supposed to Go. And I Was at My Wits End..."

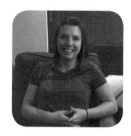 Hi, I'm Erica. I'm 24-years-old. I've been dealing with bilateral joint pain since I was 12 or 13. When I was younger, it was always because I did too many sports. Okay, chalked it up as that. I got out of high school, wasn't doing sports, but continued with joint pain, bilateral joint pain. At this point, it was in every joint in my body, my toes, my fingers, you name it, and it hurt.

Went back to the doctor, now it's because I'm not doing anything. I let it go. Now I can't sleep. I'm having headaches. I have no energy and I'm having constipation issues. I finally go back to a different physician, I get blood work drawn, and finally somebody listens to me. They start me on Methotrexate, one injection a week. I did that for about three months and it didn't do any good. We changed to tablets, sulfasalazine. I have now had to increase that two times. It still was not helping.

My lovely husband decided to look into stem cell therapy as soon as I got diagnosed last summer. At first, I was skeptical. I'm a nurse, so I think typical medicine, what I'm used to, what I know, should be able to fix this problem, mask it, I guess you could say. I know how rheumatoid arthritis is supposed to go by the book. Anyway, I'm at my wits end, still having joint pain through all of my joints, constipation to the point I'm having to take medication, and I don't know what else to do. I'm 24-years-old, you know, it's scary.

Six weeks ago, I come here and got three injections, well four injections, one in each knee, and they split one ml of stem cells and put it in the brown fat in my back. I've been sleeping better. I've had more energy. My constipation, I'm not having any issues, and my pain is practically gone. It does sound like it's too good to be true. I can't say I wouldn't disagree. That's how I felt for almost a year. It took my husband almost a year to convince me. He's let me do what I wanted to do, and it was not working.

These last six weeks was life changing. I would spend any amount of money to get the amount of relief that I've had these last six weeks. Now I'll have it for them majority of my life.

~ Erica

"My Doctors Were Saying My Knees Are Bone-on-Bone and Need Knee Replacement Surgery..."

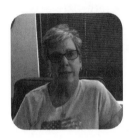 Hi, my name is Ellen. For several years now I was having knee pain. My doctors have been telling me that I'm getting bone on bone, and of course they said I'm going to need a knee replacement one day. I'm 62-years-old. I've played a lot of softball over the years. I do water skiing. I've been pretty active. I do a lot of gardening and working out in the yard, and my knees were getting progressively worse. I was getting cortisone shots, but they were getting less and less effective on me. I knew I had to do something different.

It was either go ahead and have the knee replacement, or try stem cells. I did Dr. Banerjee's stem cell program, and I'm very happy that I did. So far I'm thrilled with it. It's been wonderful for me. I could tell almost immediately that I was feeling better. After two or three days, I had less pain than I've had for the last three years. It's really been a god send for me. I'd recommend it to anyone.

My knees would be in so much pain. I'd say up to an eight, sometimes worse. It would just be miserable for me. I couldn't walk. To walk out in the yard on uneven ground, or work in my garden was just killing me. It was making me upset and depressed because this was something I loved to do.

Now, on most days I have zero pain. My pain level is nothing. It's been wonderful.

~ Ellen

"I Would Wake Up in the Morning Dreading Getting Out of Bed Because it Hurt. Dreading Having to Go to Work Because I Could Hardly Walk..."

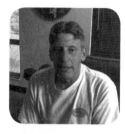

Hi, I'm Brett. I'm 55-years-old. I was probably a little skeptical like you might be. If you have arthritis in your joints and you want to be pain-free, this is the way to go. Six weeks ago I had an injection and today I'm completely pain-free. I don't take any medications for pain. I was a little apprehensive at first, but it's the best money I've spent in a long time.

I can squat down now, and get back up. I can lift my leg. I can almost run and it's only been six weeks. It is truly life changing results. It's that simple.

Before my stem cell therapy, I would wake up in the morning dreading getting out of bed because it hurt. Dreading having to go to work because I could hardly walk. I'm a maintenance guy and there's a lot of walking involved, a lot of getting down on my knees working on my equipment, machinery.

I can do all that now. I've had zero pain medication. No Aleve, no Naproxen, no Percocet, no nothing. It's truly life changing, honest to go god. God has also been a part of that. He led me to Dr. Banerjee, and it's worked 100% for me.

~ Brett

"I Couldn't Sleep Because of the Constant Pain in My Feet, and Neuropathy..."

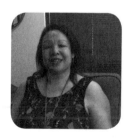

Hi, I'm Vivi. I've been with Dr. Banerjee since August 23rd with my first procedure. I am just really thrilled because I had a lot of pain from a car accident January 5th, 2012. I was in constant pain and I couldn't sleep because of the constant pain in my feet, and some neuropathy. I couldn't really move my toes or ankles, and I have plantar fasciitis in the right foot. I had a fifth metatarsal Jones break in the left foot.

What happened is, it's been a little over a month since August 23rd, and I'm on my first follow-up with Dr. Banerjee. I can sleep now because I have no chronic pain in my feet. I can move my toes and I can move my ankles. I'm just thrilled to tears. I'm telling everyone, my family and friends, they have got to do this.

The pain scale was about a nine. It would keep me up, I couldn't sleep. It was constant. It was very painful to walk. Now, it's zero. Two injections. I had 1cc in one ankle, and another 1cc in the other ankle as far as the shot. I'm telling you, it's been miraculous. I could start move my toes even immediately after the shots. I can't believe this, but I'm telling everyone!

~ Vivi

"I Have Had Nine Knee Surgeries..."

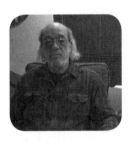

My name's Amos and I'm 63-years-old. I've already had nine knee surgeries. I had seven on my right leg, in which they replaced my knee in September of 2014, which they went back in and redid in November of 2014, in which he messed it all up because it hyper extends on me. On my left leg, I've had two knee surgeries already on it, arthroscopy. I had a shot in my left knee, stem cell shot, about seven weeks ago. Since then, I'm able to squat down and stand back up without pain in my left knee. Still in my right knee, but none in my left knee.

My clicking in my knee, isn't like it used to be. It's getting so much better already. The knee basically has tightened up for me. It's the best thing I've done. I spend $20,000 plus with insurance on my right knee, and I wouldn't sell it to nobody for a nickel.

On my left knee, I went and took a stem cell shot in it, and it's the best thing I've ever done in my life. I'm very, very happy. I would recommend this to everybody. I hope that everyone could have the same success that I have. If you don't believe me, ask my wife. She's very, very happy about the difference that she has seen in me.

It's nice to be able to go out and walk up and down the steps, and not have the pain and all that that I've dealt with for many years. Now I can squat all the way down, and I can squat all the way back up. I don't feel it in this knee. I still feel it in my fake knee.

Best thing I ever done in my life. I don't have to go to therapy. I spent hundreds of hours of therapy and weeks of therapy with all the operations I had before. There isn't any therapy in this.

~ Amos

"My Pain Scale Was a 10, I Could Hardly Walk..."

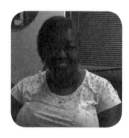 My name is Anne. I am 61. Prior to stem cell therapy I had trouble with my left knee, my hips would feel like they were kind of burning like they just had a really tough workout. They would be tired. My lower back hurt when I would stand for more than 10 or 15 minutes, and I would have to find somewhere to sit down.

After my stem cell therapy, my knee feels a lot better. I haven't used any Advil, or Tylenol, or anything. I pivoted, it would just really hurt. It would be so sore. Now, I can pivot and walk without any pain. It's pretty good.

I haven't had any problems with my hips, and my lower back is feeling a lot better. I had one injection in my knee. It's been about six weeks, so I see a noticeable improvement. The pain scale in my knee was about, I would have given it a 10, because I could hardly pivot or walk without any pain. I would kind of hop around. I would have to take something to relieve the pain, some Advil or something. Now, I notice that I don't have to do that. I do walk a lot better. Now I would give it, I would say about a three. I've also lost about seven pounds since the last six weeks. I'm happy with it. I'm pleased.

~ Ann

"I Couldn't Stand For More Than Five Minutes..."

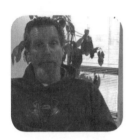

My name is Clarence. I had the stem cells in my back. I couldn't hardly stand for over five minutes. Since I had the stem cells, I'm able to get around, move a lot better than I could before. I can stand for more than five minutes without sitting down. I notice a considerable improvement within two weeks of the stem cells. Now I'm at six weeks right now, and I'm feeling really good. Highly recommend it, recommend it to about six different people so far.

~ Clarence

"If You Have Tried Everything Else and Nothing Has Worked, Try Stem Cells..."

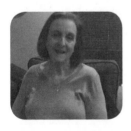

My name is Diane. I'm 64-years-old. I have AFib, so I can't take any Advil, or Aleve, or anything like that. I can only take Tylenol for pain. I have osteoarthritis. I went to a seminar, and then I came in and spoke to Dr. Banerjee. I decided, I'm going to try this. I've tried everything else.

I came in and I got five injections. I had each hand done. I had my left hip, my left knee, and my right ankle. After the first injection on my hand, my left hand, I merely felt a warm sensation go to my elbow. I guess that was the stem cell. Within just a few minutes I was able to snap my fingers. I have not been able to snap my fingers on this hand in probably seven years. They said, "Don't get too excited, don't do that. Just relax and let us finish our treatment."

After all the treatment was done, I went home and just relaxed. My husband later said, "Look at your ankles." I'm like, "Oh great, now what?" He said, "They're not swollen." They have been swollen for years. That night, I got myself in bed with my hands behind my back. I haven't done that in probably six years. I didn't even have a shot in my shoulder, so that was a free benefit.

My hands, all my knuckles have hurt for years with the arthritis. They don't hurt anymore.

I was skeptical at first, but I'm telling you, it works. If you have tried everything else and nothing has worked, try stem cells, because it's worth it. My knees used hurt so bad; I would have to support myself to get up with my hands. Now I can jump up without having pain on my knees.

I would say before stem cell therapy my pain level was a 10, and now probably, I don't know, two or three on a bad day. My right ankle would hurt and I would limp. People would always say, "Oh what's wrong, you're limping?" I'm like, "I am?" I didn't even know I limped because it hurt so bad. I don't have people asking me why I'm limping.

My pain level is probably, I don't know, maybe a two. I don't even recognize I'm having pain. My left hip used to wake me up in the night because it would hurt so bad, and I couldn't sleep on my left side for anything. Now I find myself waking up on my left side.

I don't really think I have a lot of pain anymore. I would recommend it for anybody. I've referred it to a lot of people. I'm saying, instead of taking a lot of medicine, and don't have surgery, try this first, it's worth your money to try it.

~ Dianne

"I Knew Surgery Was Not The Way I Wanted To Be Healing Myself..."

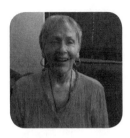

In my line of work I've seen a lot of people returning for repeat surgeries on their shoulders and their knees. When I started having issues in my shoulders and my knees, I knew surgery was not the way I wanted to be healing myself. When I saw a video on the stem cell, I knew that this was for me. After my stem cell therapy my issues with my knees and left shoulder are resolved.

Dr. Banerjee's videos on the self-healing techniques, like the tapping, the castor oil packs, the cooking appropriately, eating the healthy foods, healthy menus, those have all been very helpful. His stem cell enhancement program was very beneficial.

I absolutely would recommend stem cells to anybody. They can't do anything but help you heal.

~ Evelon

"Now I'm Living It to the Fullest Extent. I Feel Younger Even In My Activity..."

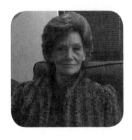

I'm Hazel and I'm 75-years-old. I've really enjoyed the last few months, because before the last months, I would have a hard time walking. I would spend a lot of time in the chair with my legs wrapped up with the heating blanket. I felt like I was wasting time. When I would get up and walk on them, and then I would go back to my chair.

Since having the stem cells, I've been able to do a lot more outside. We have three acres, and gardening, doing that, enjoying it, before it was painful to do it. Since having the stem cell, I've had a lot more mobility. My daughter asked me to go to Haiti with her on a humanitarian venture, and I was able to go and keep up with the rest of the group. When she first asked if I could go, he says, "Well can she bend over and pick up stuff?" My daughter says, "Yeah, I think she can do that."

When I got over there, I kept up with the rest of the crew. They told me a number of times that they wondered how I would be do everything. I kept up with them. I entertained 40 little Haiti children and was able to have a wonderful time with them. Two days after I got back from Haiti, I went on a camp out. I do reenactments, the Lewis and Clark time period, and was there for four days, and able to keep up with the rest of the group. It was cold, but I didn't have any trouble with my legs and I just enjoyed it.

I feel younger even in my activity. I was thinking I was just going to be sitting in my chair for a long time, until I decided to check out. Now I am Living it to the fullest extent. Recommend Dr. Banerjee's stem cell program highly. Highly recommend it. Check into it. Find out about it. That'll put you on the right track. Sorry. We are blessed to have this technology.

~ Hazel

"Within 24 Hours Literally, My Knee Pain Disappeared. My Sleep Got Better. My AFib Disappeared. My Blood Pressure is Back to Normal..."

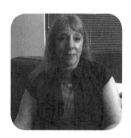

Hello, my name is Connie and I'm 70-years-old. Approximately three years ago I was having extreme pain in my left knee. I had had a meniscus tear which was repaired, but after that, very shortly after that, it just got bad again. I was becoming more and more limited in my abilities to perform normal duties, or even normal activities of daily life. In the last year, I became sedentary actually because of the pain. I knew that I was going to ultimately have to resort to having a knee surgery.

One day, out of the clear blue sky, I happened to come across a post on the internet with Dr. Banerjee talking about stem cell treatments. I thought, you know, I know that they've been working on this for a long time. I'm a retired nurse. I was a nurse for 40 years. Years and years ago, when I first started nursing, they were already talking about stem cell research, and I knew it was going to take many decades for this to be either approved, or thought as a successful way of treatment, because you need many decades to pass so your people who you experiment with giving it too, they have to have some long term results.

Anyway, after this post that I read, I decided to come to a seminar that Dr. Banerjee was giving. I was more than convinced that this was the way for me to go. I wasn't prepared to go through major surgery with possible maybe not a good outcome. Not all surgeries are successful. I went ahead and signed on, and got the cells. It was six weeks ago today actually.

I was astonished. Within 24 hours literally, my knee pain disappeared, within that week, first week, I noticed several other things that had been troubling me for so long. I had had awful pain in my shoulder and neck when I was sleeping. I had miserable nights of sleep. That had completely disappeared. I have been diagnosed with AFib, and prior to the treatment I was having shortness of breath on very little exertion, and rapid heartbeats frequently. All of those things were depressing me terribly.

Those also disappeared. My blood pressure has now turned into normal all of a sudden and I don't take any blood pressure medicines anymore. Soon, when I go to see my heart doctor, which is probably going to be several months, I'm going to see if I can just stop taking my heart medicine because I don't know why I'm taking it.

I feel good. I have a lot of energy. I feel renewed. I'm very blessed to have come across Dr. Banerjee's post, and I would recommend it to anyone. It's the wave of the future as far as I'm concerned, and also because of the past and what I know about the research. I would recommend it again to anybody, anyone suffering from any type of neurological pains, or any pains in your joints.

I mean again, I did not expect having no rapid heartbeats after this. I thought that was something just unexpectedly that happened. My energy level is very good. My sleep is really good. My energy level is tremendously different. I feel like this is a great way to go and it has improved my life. Now, instead of looking at the future as something that was going to be doomsday for me, I'm looking at it as a renewal and a way of being able to actually experience things that I probably would have not been able to do hadn't I done this.

~ Connie

"My Pain Was So Bad I Could Hardly Walk. It Gripped Me Like Vice. After I Got My Injections, The Next Day I Started Immediately Feeling Relieve..."

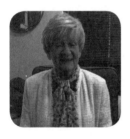 My name is Lynn and I'm 77-years-old, and I came to Dr. Banerjee about 12 weeks ago, maybe a little less. I got my injections, one half in either side of my neck, either side of my hip, and then the right side of my hip. I have cartilage losing out of my right leg, and it's because I've had damage there from many years of sports and building a home and everything.

I now don't have any pain there now. I don't have any pain in my back. I don't have any pain in my neck. My shoulder pain is less. I was getting charley horses in my right hand, and charley horses in my legs, and that has subsided. I can't say enough about the injections and I was really apprehensive.

I even had some members of my family tell me I was wasting my time. Now they're believers. I said, "It's a miracle." Now I appreciate Dr. Banerjee and all he's doing for us.

If you're doubtful, you need to come and see this for yourself. I'm a living proof. I'm not an advertisement. I'm just an ordinary American. I just praise God that I was able to find him, and he was able to find me.

I suggest anyone that's having problems, please come and at least talk to Dr. Banerjee.

My pain was so bad when I came here I could hardly walk. It gripped me like a vice. After I got my injections, the next day I started immediately feeling relieve. Then I went on Dr. Banerjee's eating plan. I stick with it pretty good. I've lost almost 20 pounds in 12 weeks, and I was not hungry. I feel so much better. I got all the poisons out of my body.

My activity is wonderful. My daughter told me the other day, she said, "Mom, you've got a spring in your step. I haven't seen that in five years." I took care of my dear sweet husband for 14 years. He had dementia. I lifted him an awful lot toward the end. I did a lot of damage to my back. Now, I'm getting stronger. I just wanted to share that with people so they can have the same health that I have today.

~ Lynn

"I Was Hurt In a Bad Car Accident. I Used to Hurt Everywhere. Would Get Up Every Morning and Be Angry at the Kid That Hit Me From Behind..."

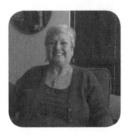

Hi, my name is Joan, I'm 68-years-old. I'm a former professional singer. I was hurt in a bad accident years ago for which there was nothing anybody could do at that time. I had stem cell therapy on Valentines Day, 2/14/2019 with Dr. Banerjee. This is something I was not able to do awhile back, for years. I also used to swing dance before I was injured. Now I can dance again. I couldn't do this at all. I couldn't bend down. I couldn't do anything.

I would get up every morning and be angry at the kid that hit me from behind. Anyway, I'm doing fine now. I'm on my way to recovery. It's only been a little over a month and I am absolutely amazed. I used to hurt everywhere. I hurt in my hips and my back, in my knees, in my foot, in my shoulders. I even had torn rotator cuffs that were just slightly torn, but I don't have any trouble with that anymore. I'm doing just great.

I had one injection, which Dr. Banerjee split in half because I was having sciatic nerve pain on both sides. He gave me half and half on each side of the number four vertebrae.

It's been wonderful. I'm very grateful. My shoulder is feeling great. I can move them all around.

I've already recommended Dr. Banerjee's stem cell program for many people. I can't tell you how many people I've sent this to and had them look at it. My little brother up in Maine was in town. He says, "I'm going to do that." He said he needed knee replacement. I said, "Oh no you don't Bill, oh no you don't. This is wonderful, try it."

~ Joan

"I Am Not Using a Walker Anymore..."

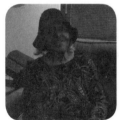

My name is Betty and I'm 83-years-old, and I have arthritis in both knees. The pain got to the point where I was on a walker. When I took the stem cell treatment, tried it, in six weeks, I wasn't using the walker anymore. Before stem cell therapy it was very painful to walk.

My right arm and my hand used to bother me. It doesn't bother me much anymore. It wasn't injected my arms.

I would recommend this for other people. Oh yeah, I would.

~ Betty

"I Can Walk better And My Shoulder Pain Doesn't Wake Me Up At Night..."

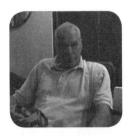

Hi, my name is Rich. I am 70-years-old and it's been six weeks now since I had the stem cell injection in my knee. I have noticed that the pain is less. I can walk better. Also, I had a shoulder pain. My left shoulder was giving me lot of problems. I couldn't sleep on it at night. I notice now that I wake up in the middle of the night, and I'm lying on my left shoulder and it's not painful as it used to be. It has been working. The pain in my knee went from about a six down to I would say now about a one. I can do more. I exercise a little bit more. It is definitely working.

~ Rich

"After My Stroke, I Had Daily Headaches For 20 Months. Within 48 Hours Of My Stem Cells My Headaches Were Gone..."

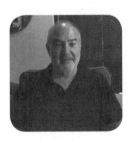

I came to get a stem cell injection for a knee pain that I had been suffering with for 45 years. It's been a good success for my knee. A side bar benefit was the fact that I had suffered a stroke in September of 2016. I had been left as a residue of the stroke, a headache that was daily, intense, some days way more than others. The headache had been with me for almost 20 months.

Within 48 hours of the stem cell injection that I received, my headache subsided. I have been headache free for six weeks. That has been an unbelievable benefit to me mentally and physically. It just is amazing what happened. My neurologist reluctantly is giving credit where credit goes. They have lowered some of the pills that they had me taking. My headaches, again, came after a stroke. There was absolutely not one thing, not one pill that helped ever.

I did not get the stem cell injection thinking it was going to help my headaches. It was amazing that that happened. I came for a knee situation and the headaches are gone. We're six weeks post stem cell injection. I am not suffering a headache this moment. I haven't had one in probably 17 days. I know it sounds funny that I know all this, but when you have a headache every day for 20 months, you know way more about it than you want to know.

My knee has responded also. I am feeling strength. I have a better start to every day. I do not wake up ever with a knee problem. When I wake up it's a new start. I compare it to hitting a reset button. My knee is in good shape to start the day. The strength in the muscles around the knee get better every day. I'm under repair.

I can do things I haven't been able to do. I don't suffer the pain that I had been suffering. I've had my knee scoped, I've had my knee treated, we're on the right path with the stem cell injection that has given me less chronic pain. It's given me pain-free movements.

I also suffered from a hand injury. My hand, around my right knuckles, was swollen, painful, it was tough to grip a golf club, grip a tool. It got worse as the years went along. Again, this isn't something that I thought, "okay I hope when they help my knee, my hand stops hurting." That did not occur to me. About 10 days ago I said to my wife, "You know, my hand isn't swollen. Did you notice that it's not swelled up?" She was like, "Well let me look at it," very surprised that the swelling in the knuckles was down.

I am very pleased. Would recommend Dr. Banerjee's stem cell program for anyone.

~ Tim

"I Needed a Hip Replacement. Now I Don't Even Need Pain Medicine..."

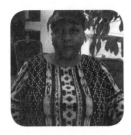

The pain has gone from a 10 to a four. My weight has decreased. My blood pressure is good. I'm just really excited. I recommend that anyone that is interested in doing it, they should take the chance. I needed a hip replaced in both hips. Now I'm able to move around. I'm not taking any pain medicine since I've completed the stem cells. I would recommend it.

~ Sherri

"My Doctors Told Me I Had Suicide Pain..."

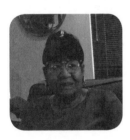

I was in severe pain all 2017 and 20018 winter. It seemed like I lived at the emergency room every night. I have reduced all the pain down the left side of my body by having stem cell injections. I can walk. I can wear my heels again. I can resume some of my housework and my yard work. I feel much better.

My pain level was all the way to 10. Some of my pain I had, my doctors would call it suicide pain, that's how bad it was. I couldn't walk. I couldn't go to the bathroom. I couldn't dress myself. I couldn't do anything until I had a stem cell injection. I got one injection divided into half on each side of my body. The left side was the worst side, so they put left and right side, so I wouldn't favor my right side.

When I first got the injection, I walked out the door and I noticed a difference. I couldn't sleep at night before. I noticed that I wasn't bending over in the morning. I wasn't tossing and turning all night. I just noticed a difference, and I could tell that I was trying to get back to my normal activities. It got better and better. I'm 30 days in, so I feel much better. Oh, I'm trying to tell all my friends. It's a miracle.

~ Janis

Table of Contents

Why Your Health Matters

Let's Choose a Healing Journey That Focuses on YOU!

The decision to begin your journey to recovery is yours and yours alone. If you choose to focus on your healing, that can start right here. Making the shift can be intimidating, and often the pain can cloud what we think we are capable of.

That is why my team and I do what we do. We care about your health. We want to lead you through a healing journey, so you can get back to enjoying life and doing what you love to do.

Without your health, you have nothing—your life becomes limited to what you are capable of doing, not what you truly want to do, and to how long you can persevere through your daily tasks. I see patients whose health has become a steady decline. It is torturous to see anyone go through that.

For many people, their daily activities can be a challenge, and tasks that give a person freedom to live independently are restricted—things like these:

- Playing with your grandkids
- Having all the energy you desire
- Doing all your favorite activities like hiking or golfing
- Climbing up and down stairs
- Getting dressed
- Walking or dancing
- Staying awake all day

- Opening jars, or other tasks that require twisting
- Going out with friends
- Traveling

Although they may be minute details most healthy people do not think about, losing the ability to accomplish these tasks is losing freedom. To make matters worse, as physical ability declines, people are obviously less active, which also means they are not able to exercise, and it becomes a downward spiral.

Sometimes, when you witness people experiencing chronic pain, or you go through it yourself, you feel so helpless and out of control. It is awful to watch someone die of a degenerative condition in front of your eyes and not be able to do anything about it.

That is why I care about your health! Too many of my loved ones suffered before I saw there is a different way. Then I went to the experts and studied it, getting firsthand experience in how stem cell therapy is working on real people, every day.

If you want a better life for yourself, I invite you to take steps today, beginning with understanding how your health is being impacted by your condition. Do you accept the invitation? Are you ready to focus on what really matters?

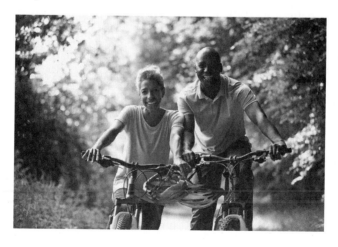

Regeneration: The Road to Healing

Your health is why I am doing this. As I watched family members and patients suffer in pain, I became relentless in my search for a way to help. And I knew that the way I could help people had to go beyond traditional treatments. People are used to the medical system, so when it fails them, they are unsure of what to do next.

Usually, as we will discuss more deeply when I go into some of the specifics about each condition, there is a standard treatment and procedure that occurs. Unfortunately, the standard is not good enough, and in a lot of cases, it is masking the symptoms and making the condition worse.

Regardless of what is wrong with a patient, the process usually looks something like this:

1. **Diagnosis:** Finding out what is wrong happens through a combination of patient history, doctor examination, and blood or urine testing.
2. **Further Testing:** To pinpoint the specifics of the condition on that patient, more testing is done. This can include X-ray, MRI, or other imaging tests, further bloodwork, or a host of other options.
3. **Treatment:** Medication is prescribed to subdue symptoms. So whatever problems the condition is causing, be it pain, immobility, heartburn, high blood pressure, you name it, doctors can prescribe something to relieve those symptoms. Of course, this does nothing to heal the patient or treat the condition. It is usually a stop-gap measure to maintain a certain quality of life.
4. **Surgery:** When a condition worsens, and depending on the results of the testing, surgery might be optional or required. Surgery can repair broken bones and fix other damaged tissue

and organs. It also comes with complications, and often, recovery time can be quite lengthy.

5. **Monitoring the Condition:** Requiring frequent follow-up with medical professionals, many conditions must be closely monitored as they progress. Especially with degenerative conditions, the only option sometimes is to watch patients lose their health.

It breaks my heart how many people come to me, basically hopeless. The thing is, they want more for themselves, or they wouldn't be here. The question is, do you want more for yourself?

Choosing to Live a Better Life

So many people want a better life. They often feel like they have run out of options and have no hope left. When, in fact, they just haven't heard all of the available information yet, or been given options outside the realm of mainstream medicine.

For many people, they still have time to make the decision to seek out answers. It comes down to not allowing someone, even a doctor, to take away your hope. Through this book, we are going to try to bring back some of that hope.

My job is educating you, to allow you to make the best decisions to help your body heal. It is a process that allows us to find out what is causing your pain and implement a therapy that promotes regeneration. In essence, it is about helping you be your best self.

This is not about making any promises for quick-health, miracle fixes, even if some of our patient's testimonials suggest otherwise. I take a focused approach to your body's natural healing tendencies and use scientific knowledge of cell function to boost that healing.

I like to think of it as boosting your healing potential, and it is there for anyone seeking help. So many of my patients have very different conditions and issues that lead them to seek help. Others might have more than one issue from my long list of usual suspects.

The list, included in a shortened version here, shows the broad symptoms from the tip of the head to the bottom of the foot and everywhere in between. So many people are not getting healed because they do not know that stem cell therapy can improve the following conditions:

- Knee pain
- Skin trauma and wound healing
- Joint problems
- Hip Pain
- Cardiovascular issues
- Inflammation
- Diabetes
- Shoulder Pain
- Thyroid issues
- Arthritis
- Chronic fatigue
- Autoimmune deficiency
- Kidney function issues
- Spinal cord injury
- Nerve damage and disorders

As a doctor of natural medicine, I have been helping patients with these conditions and more—some of which had not even been diagnosed—for two decades. Here is the thing, I just want you to feel better and have a better quality of life.

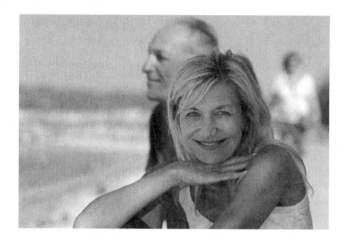

Why I Chose to Offer Stem Cell Therapy

In the next few pages, I am going to share my real *why*—the story that I see in the eyes of every patient I meet. See, it is personal, and I see everyone as an earlier version of my aunt who died tragically and unnecessarily.

I believe with all my heart that if she had had stem cell therapy, she would be alive today, and so, I will share her story soon. Before we lost her, I had a completely different view of the medical system. It took some extreme circumstances, but I learned about health in a way that I had never been taught before.

As a doctor, I was taught to trust the science. It was only when a health-care crisis hit close to home that I realized our medical system is not doing that. Not by a long shot. Instead, they are making money by prolonging people's conditions instead of healing them.

So when I came across stem cell therapy, I followed the studies and read the research, and it clicked. Then, I heard patient testimonials and saw the procedure in person, and the results were undeniable.

There is so much information and science that I have studied and will continue to study about how the human body works and how its systems promote healing.

People often ask why I choose to offer stem cell therapy since it is a new and sometimes controversial option. After telling them that stem cell therapy has been around for quite a while and is scientifically proven, I give them my answer. There are many reasons, but these are my top three:

1. **Noninvasive:** Most of my patients have had enough pain to last multiple lifetimes. Offering a solution that is fast and pain-free with little to no risk is a relief to them, as it is to me as their caregiver.

2. **Natural Healing:** Stem cell therapy uses the body's natural systems to promote   regeneration and healing.

3. **Results Driven:** Every patient who comes back to me with a smile is my why. I got so tired of witnessing people suffer, and now, I get to be a big part of their healing breakthrough.

The combination of the safety and regulation of the procedure, along with the proven ongoing health benefits, makes stem cell therapy a no-brainer.

My Objectives and Promise to You

This information is here to give patients an understanding of their conditions, as well as options that have been successful for many others—and hope to get the results they long for. When patients come in to speak with me, I treat them like my family. They are important to me—as if I were treating my own mom.

Now I want to extend that level of caring into this book, so I can reach everyone, even if I cannot meet them face to face. You can be assured that the information in this book is based on my knowledge, experience, training with other doctors, and clinical trials. Everything contained here is what I tell my patients when they come to me.

Lately, I have realized how important it is for patients to have access to information. Instead of giving blanket statements or providing no recourse, as doctors, it is our duty to encourage patients to seek out all possible options on their healing journey. If I can help my patients live the life they want to live, that is my overall objective—whether they spend one dime with me or not. For too many years, I have watched patients with such bad degeneration in their lives, and all their doctors were recommending was surgery or pain medications.

My promise to my patients is that I will:

- Always continue learning about their condition and how to heal it.
- Work with experts in the field to provide the best options for my patients.
- Study the research behind stem cell therapy for the most advanced knowledge.
- Be open and honest with my patients throughout all encounters.
- Maintain a professional and comfortable environment.
- Provide multiple options for an overall healthier life.

I don't want anyone to be on drugs or in pain. This is why I brought stem cells into my practice. I had a great practice—but people were still needing help. Stem cell therapy is just one more way to help people and give them back their quality of life.

There are thousands and thousands of people all around us struggling to maintain a normal quality of life. These people are not living, they are merely existing, and they are who I want to reach most.

*"It is not the years in your life, but the
life in your years that counts."*

~ Adlai Stevenson

By putting it all together in book form, I hope the information will pass from person to person to reach those most vulnerable and in need of help. For anyone who has had to watch a loved one go through the struggles of chronic conditions, know that there may well be a better way.

I am going to share the story of my own mom, because her story is a mirror image to that of so many thousands of other moms who suffer with diabetes. People are getting blood tests done to measure their blood sugar levels, and they are typically given medication and a pamphlet on exercise and eating properly. But it goes far beyond that. Although there are so many other ways to help patients with diabetes get control of their health, outdated medical practices are still in place, and the time is not taken to dig deeper into the problem. The truth is there are some very practical steps that can be taken to greatly improve the quality of life for the patient.

My Mom

Almost every patient I see reminds me of my mom in one way or another. All of them share something similar to what she went through, struggling to find answers. Struggling also to cope with a body that was slowly failing her. For far too many years, I saw my mom get sicker and sicker, and suffer as no person should. It ripped my heart to pieces and devastated our entire family. It also had a profound, long-lasting impact on how I practice health care. My patient's health became much more personal.

Years ago, when I first had a chiropractic practice, a few years after I had graduated, my mom was going through some health issues. She had been recently diagnosed with diabetes and had been suffering from extreme fatigue. At the time, I lived a few hours away and would go to see my mom for the weekend about once a month. Whenever I arrived, Mom would try to hide her sickness, but it became more and more obvious she was not doing well.

Every few months, she would get another viral or bacterial infection that seemed to really wear her down. On top of that, her joints were bothering her, and she had debilitating neck pain. Although she took medication for the pain, it didn't seem to help. Whenever something new came up, she was given more pills to take indefinitely. There she was, going from doctor to doctor, and they would placate her by telling her about different test results, all of which were irrelevant because it wasn't helping her.

My mom believed in doctors at the time, trusting they had all the information she needed. There were times when she had to wait months or years for the new pills to do their work, and still she saw no improvement in how she felt. She wouldn't let anyone touch her, and all her other muscles and joints were starting to feel the stress of her condition. Her neck pain became so bad that she felt like someone was pouring hot coals on her neck, and the burning nerve pain intensified.

Every time the doctor prescribed something new, she took it as directed without receiving an explanation as to what it was. One day, she came home with a bag full of pills. No one could tell her why she was still in so much pain, and doctors often suggested that it might be all in her head.

I got fed up. I started doing my own research and contacting doctors who were claiming to be reversing diabetes. I read books, and then contacted the authors to learn from them. Then I took what I learned from them, and I used it to help my mom.

She was a tough patient, and both my parents were skeptical because they trusted the medical community. Eventually though, we managed to reverse some of her symptoms. Within six months of changing my mom's treatment, we saw these improvements:

- Blood pressure reduced
- Lower blood sugar
- Increased energy
- Less irritability/anxiousness
- Healed joint and nerve pain

She was a changed woman. Every day, she gained more energy. As her pain went down, she was able to do more throughout the day and didn't feel like she was living on edge. She was elated and felt like she had been given a second chance at life.

It took me longer to win over my father. He is an old-fashioned guy, and he thought the doctors knew what was best for his wife. Still, as my mom's numbers improved, and she started to feel better, their confidence in what I was doing increased. Eventually, my dad couldn't believe the difference in her condition that came about from what we did.

At the same time, they were shocked, angered, and saddened at what they learned through the process. My mom was devastated to think how her own sister could have been saved, if only we had this knowledge a little earlier.

Family Comes First—My Aunt's Story

I am also going to share the story of my aunt, because it is an important story to tell. I just wish I could have lived closer to her to see what really was going on. Knowing what I know now, her story could have had a very different ending.

She meant a lot to me and was around my whole life. My mom considered my aunt her best friend, and they were so similar in a lot of ways, especially when it came to their health. They both started to experience similar symptoms of diabetes around the same time. Though my aunt did seem much worse than my mom. She reacted poorly to medication, and her health declined more rapidly.

My aunt died a slow, painful death at age fifty-two. It was labeled as a diabetic stroke, but more likely, it was caused by the cocktails of medications prescribed to her for years on end. Yet no one even looked further into her death. And it turned out, no one was really looking after her while she was alive. When I found out the doctors had given my aunt the incorrect information, I knew she should not have died. I also knew I had to find a better way for people. One that did not lead to a negative outcome, so agonizing and drawn out.

So I sought out the information I have to offer you, and I didn't stop until I had a solid base. My family's story inspired me to help others and share this information. I must keep sharing this knowledge and offering treatments so that people can find hope for a future with their loved ones, instead of having to find how to go on without them.

So, Who Am I?

I am Dr. Raj Banerjee, a leading expert on health and wellness in St. Louis, Missouri. My health-care clinic, called Integrative Health Care of St. Louis, LLC, has been in practice for well over a decade, helping patients find healing and recovery from a whole-health perspective, and offering options unavailable to them in the mainstream medical system.

Working with each individual patient, I specialize in customizing natural-treatment programs, targeting an array of health issues. Since

I started, I have used this approach to aid in the recovery and healing from these conditions:

- Thyroid issues
- Adrenal fatigue
- Belly fat and weight issues
- Autoimmune disease
- Diabetes
- Food cravings
- Depression
- Fatigue
- Cardiovascular disorders
- Hormone imbalances
- Fibromyalgia
- Chronic fatigue syndrome
- Joint pain
- Many other common health complaints

My ongoing training and education includes a doctorate in Chiropractic from Logan College. I have broad experience in various approaches to creating hormonal and spinal balance. Using this knowledge and experience, I have tutored students and other doctors on the Liebenson's protocol for rehabilitation.

In addition to my active practice, I spend a lot of time speaking at seminars and helping people make positive changes in their lives. To share my information and resources, I offer lab-based assessments and specific lifestyle programing. Also, I have authored two books as well as online programs about health and healing.

It is my passion to make sure as many people as possible know more about their pathways to healing. Through all of this, and especially when I meet with a patient one-on-one, I tailor these treatment programs to include a focus on the following bodily processes:

- Hormonal
- Immune
- Digestive
- Detoxification
- Cardiovascular

The aim is to give the systems of the body an overall approach to wellness. What we must do is look at each patient's specific and individual needs, and then create a customized treatment protocol for that individual. In the end, I am here to serve you and to be a source of information and support to those who suffer needlessly.

This Is about Healing You!

By now, I hope you know there is hope. You can have an improved quality of life and you can find out what options are best for your health condition. By your reading through this book, much of that will be revealed to you.

To be effective and efficient in disseminating this information for each individual reader, I will divide medical conditions into easy to follow sections, so each person can read what is personally relevant.

My goal here is for you to be informed, for you to learn about a health therapy, using stem cells, that, through research study and scientific experimentation, is showing success after success. Through the information I present and the testimonials you will read, I want you to have a better understanding of this approach to treatment and to be comfortable enough to consider it as an option for your own health.

It warms my heart to see people get healthy. I don't want any more families going through what mine did when we lost my aunt. It is just so hard and, often, so unnecessary. So take what you can from these words, and regardless of what else happens, use it as a starting point for a better life.

It Is Time to Take Matters into Your Own Hands

Though regenerative medicine and stem cell therapy is new to most people, it has been around for quite awhile and is becoming more and more often, the least invasive and most beneficial option for many different patients. So let's find out why.

While you read this book, through each chapter, patient story, and research discussion, keep yourself in mind. How does it relate to you and your situation? Focus on your health and healing, and see if any of this resonates with you.

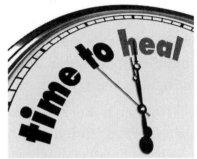

You know yourself and the effects your condition is having on you better than anyone else.

Too often, doctors read about a condition or study it only briefly in medical school, but they do not know or understand what it is like to live with the condition. And for some rarer disorders, they probably spent minimal time studying it.

So, if you agree to the following statements, get ready to change your life by improving your health:

- Focusing on my health takes all my energy.
- With so much contradictory information about my condition, I don't know where to turn or whom to trust.
- So many offering health treatments make promises, but don't explain why or how they work.
- I want to feel better, but I struggle just to make it through the day.
- If only I could heal as quickly as I could ten or fifteen years ago.

Most people find, like I did, that stem cell therapy offers a chance of a lifetime that can make a significant difference in the quality of life you experience.

This Is an Invitation to Change Your Life!

I invite you to keep an open mind, do your own research, come to a live seminar, and get your questions answered. Our health is our greatest asset, and it is not something we can take lightly. Pain is a terrible thing to live with, but with the advancements in medical treatments, there are options to give you the life you want to live.

Nothing is more satisfying to me than seeing a patient become pain-free and relish how their own body was able to heal. I want to be a part of your truly enjoying your life, spending more time doing the things you love to do, and enjoying quality time with friends and family.

Whatever you do, don't stop looking for answers. Learn about your health and condition and be your best advocate. Have hope—it is time to heal.

CHAPTER 1

Introduction to Stem Cells

Embracing a New Healing Option

New technology and therapies that are not well understood can make people uncertain. At the same time, procedures that are not well understood often become controversial with much misinformation being shared. So how can you embrace a new healing option if you are not sure how to gauge its accuracy?

Stem cell therapies fit in the category of "controversial" because, even though they have been used for health and wellness purposes for close to a decade, these are relatively new procedures. Nonetheless, the results some people have obtained are becoming too significant to ignore.

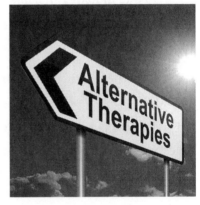

Use of the scientific method has resulted in research studies providing accurate information about the nature of the healing power of stem cells.

More and more, you are hearing doctors talk about the efficacy of stem cells. It comes as a surprise to many that stem cell therapies have been clinically proven time and again.

It is only in recent years that the positive benefits of stem cell therapy are becoming more well known. Because knowledge is the key to success in health and in life, I want you to take the information I am about to share and use it to better your health.

Stem cells are already being used in some instances in the mainstream medical world. When an organ transplant is rejected by a person's body, the patient is given stem cells to encourage regeneration. But that is just the beginning of what stem cells are being used for. So let's get right into the heart of the information.

You might be asking yourself these questions:

1. What are stem cell therapies?
2. What results are people experiencing after undergoing stem cell therapy?
3. Who is choosing this as a health option?
4. How do you know what to expect?
5. What conditions can benefit?
6. What is the procedure and downtime?

All of these are valid concerns that we will go through using scientific resources and research into previous patients' experiences.

As medical practices evolve, it is becoming clear that stem cell therapy and regenerative medicine is fast becoming the future—where health care is headed. The more people who experience healing and improvement and the more doctors who embrace alternative healing therapies, the better off we all will be.

Every single person has unique health challenges, and part of embracing a new healing option is being open to unique solutions. Thankfully, people are becoming outspoken about the benefits they are experiencing, and regenerative medicine is being made more available because people are willing to share their experiences.

Mel Gibson is one of the first celebrities to vocalize support for stem cell therapy.[1] Going as far as to purposely discuss it in media interviews, he describes how it has changed the life of multiple people in his family. Initially, he investigated the topic due to his father's declining health. At age ninety-two, his dad had a bad hip and multiple problems common for someone his age. So he brought his father to one of the top medical facilities in the United States, and they went over his whole medical history. They listed everything that was going on, and suggested a hip replacement was necessary.

At any age, surgery can be difficult, but Mel Gibson was worried that, at ninety-two, his father would not recover well from major surgery. But he did not seem to have any other choice. His brother suggested stem cells, and he was wary. Of course, there is a lot of controversy, and traditional medical practitioners wanted nothing to do with it, voicing negative comments about even suggesting the possibility.

When the initial assessment was being done, and questions were being asked, the doctors were a little shocked to hear that at age ninety-two, Mel's dad was not taking any medication. He explained he was not on any medication because he tried to stay away from doctors and hospitals.

Eventually, after extensive study, Mel took his dad down to Panama, and he got stem cells injected in his hip. Panama is one of the few places that has laws allowing stem cell therapy and regulates ethical procedures. The clinic was hesitant, because when he got there he was not in great shape. He was in a wheelchair and not talking much. It took him awhile to even get permission to fly down there. When they finally got him there, he was given stem cell injections directly to the hip.

---

[1]   Mel Gibson on Stem Cell Therapy https://www.youtube.com/watch?v=dmd7-KjE62o

His kidneys, heart, and cells began to regenerate, and the therapy helped decrease inflammation. He got a new lease on life. He had less pain, and he could walk again. He felt improvement in many different areas of his health. It was a feeling of regeneration and energy, and he was tremendously impressed to the point where Mel Gibson wanted to share his remarkable experience, as testimony to the possibilities for stem cell therapy.

Being so well known, Mel Gibson's sharing of his story, along with the words of other patients, doctors, and caregivers is bringing stem cell therapy out from a cloud of doubt. The common thread in all these stories is that these patients and their families and friends around them were determined to find a way to better health.

Each person must make the decision to seek out answers and take control of their own healing. If your current doctor isn't doing it for you, take matters into your own hands. There are doctors who care about you and want to help, so don't settle for anything less.

If your current condition is preventing you from doing things you love with the people you love, it is time to do something different. If your life is ruled by a schedule of pills or pain management therapies, follow a different path instead, one of permanent dedication to health improvement.

What it really comes down to is how you want to live your last ten, twenty, or thirty-plus years. You can choose to let your condition dictate it for you or you can make changes now. It is up to you to decide.

Do you want to?

- Play with your grandchildren . . . or sit on the sidelines?
- Travel and go on adventures . . . or struggle to accomplish daily tasks?

- Be strong enough to enjoy your passions . . . or give in to chronic pain?
- Embrace a life of hope . . . or live with restrictions?
- Grow old with vitality . . . or wither from disease?
- Remain independent . . . or require help for everything?
- Stay active and mobile . . . or be restricted to mobility devices or bed?
- Live a holistic, health-based existence . . . or be reliant on prescriptions?
- Have a simple in-office procedure . . . or undergo major surgery?

It is your choice, and there are people ready to help you, whatever you decide. Stem cell therapy may be a great option for you. You might find your story so closely resembles one of the success stories I will share that you could have written it yourself. We get that a lot. So many patients explain how skeptical they were, until they heard someone else's experience.

The best thing you can do for yourself is to be open to learning about stem cell therapy, and that is what this book is all about. Throughout each chapter, I will offer simple examples and straight forward facts for people looking for more information. Sharing the stories of clients who have had stem cell therapy will illustrate the many different conditions and situations that have benefited from stem cell therapy. For privacy, I have changed their names, but I have tried to keep their stories intact to share the personal impact of each condition.

When it comes down to it, for me, it is all about my patients and all people who have run out of options and might be looking for something different. If nothing else, they might learn more specifically how their conditions are affecting their bodies. From there, they can work toward healing options that fit them best.

How Has Your Condition Affected Your Life?

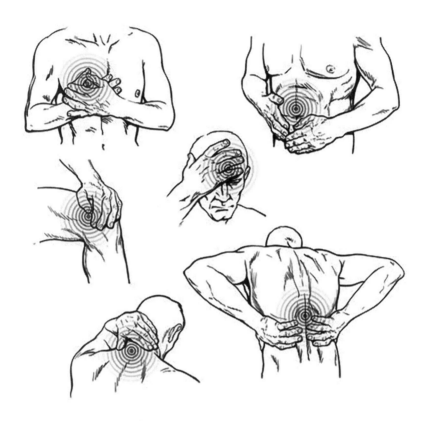

Regardless of what you already know about stem cells, I am going to walk you through the basics—from what they are, to what they do, and where they come from. We will cover it all.

But it is kind of irrelevant to some degree, right?

For the same reason we go to doctors for a quick-fix medication or cure for our conditions, we do not always want to know the exact in-and-out details of how a therapy makes us feel better.

You just want to feel better. Now this is not a lack of interest in learning; it is usually desperation.

When you are in panic mode with chronic pain or a debilitating condition, there is no room for extra information. You just cannot process it. Your body is crying out for help, and you simply rely on whatever relief can be found.

How your condition is affecting your life is too broad of an idea for most people, because it is all-consuming. Chronic pain takes over and makes everything else unimportant. When going to the bathroom, dressing, cleaning, and feeding yourself, if you have chronic pain, you may not have much energy or ability left, making it hard to focus.

As time progresses, patients become numb, and losing hope is very common. It becomes an expectation that this state is their new normal. Some people, though, refuse to give up, and these are the ones who usually make their way to me. When patients come to me, they are looking for real help. Many of them are facing surgery, or multiple surgeries, or they have given up and are barely existing, unable to move or get out and enjoy their lives in any way.

One of the reasons I became a doctor was that I have a genuine desire to help people. I want to educate people about health and see them participate in their own healing journey. I love to see people who were once very sick become vibrant and enjoy life—once more, doing the things they love most. I see stem cells as one of the best options to get patients healthy faster.

You might have come here to read about possible relief for any number of ailments. Perhaps you have heard that stem cell therapy was a viable option to improve certain conditions. Although it is easy to label a condition, we all know that the impact of the condition is way more far-reaching than that. So often, the symptoms and side effects of these conditions affect a person's entire life, making difficult, even the simplest of daily tasks.

As you read, keep in mind that, while we talk about the following specific conditions, what we are really trying to improve is *quality of life* for people who are dealing with the associated chronic pain:

- Arthritis
- Autoimmune condition
- Inflammation
- Knee pain
- Degenerative joints
- Irritable bowel syndrome (IBS)
- Parkinson's
- Spinal cord injury
- Stroke, brain injury
- Hip pain
- Cardiovascular Issues
- Tissue damage
- Long-term sports injuries
- Kidney function
- Diabetes
- Nerve Damage

Since each condition has different causes and outcomes, it is amazing to see how versatile stem cell therapy is. The study and research and years of trials are paving the way for a new form of health care that focuses on the body's ability to regenerate. Healing goes beyond all of the intricacies of these individual conditions. How your life is affected by your condition can be extremely uncomfortable. Some people find that they lose the ability to function at a normal level, as they spend their days managing symptoms of their conditions.

Mary's Story—Multiple Knee Surgeries

"Before I even heard of stem cells, I'd already had three knee surgeries. After the third time, as I was recovering from surgery, I reflected on everything else I had already tried. The meniscal tear in my knee was practically bone on bone, and the Synvisc, cortisone, and other pain medications did nothing to help.

"When I began to feel worse, after the third surgery, I also began to feel helpless. Whenever I walked, it was with a limp and excruciating pain. I couldn't move very quickly or even walk up a hill.

"Finally, my sister encouraged me to look for any other options. She did not think another surgery was going to be of any benefit to me. And in the back of my mind, I agreed, but I was terrified of having to live the rest of my life in pain and misery.

"What pushed me over the edge is when I was told that even if I did get a knee replacement, I would still have to get it redone in less than ten years. That did not seem like a pathway to healing, more like a road to more misery.

"Really, I had all but given up. Just getting through the day was exhausting, but my sister kept at me to look into this, that, and the other thing. When she mentioned stem cell therapy, it did not register right away, and then later that same day, there was a doctor on television talking about it. So I took that as a sign, at least, to find out more about it.

"At the same time, I met with my surgeon for the knee replacement that was his last-ditch effort to repair my damaged knee. It didn't

go well. He brushed off my concerns when I told him I was worried about long-term effects including these:

- *Limping*
- *Inflammation*
- *Restricted movement*
- *Chronic pain*
- *Infection and other risks associated with surgery*

"What's more is I really did not see it as a viable option because it was not a permanent fix. I believed in the power of my body to heal itself, but even this seemed like it was too late for me. I was not as young as I used to be, and my body just didn't bounce back like it used to.

"I felt like I was out of options and out of time. Recently, I had been told my knee was practically bone on bone, and a replacement was the only thing that gave me a chance to get back to my active life and start traveling again. So the surgery was scheduled.

"Now about a week before my surgery was due, I met an acquaintance who brought up stem cell therapy, and I started to do some research. It was not at all what I expected, so I postponed the surgery and went for stem cell therapy instead.

"It was the best decision I ever made. Immediately after receiving the stem cells, I felt relief from the bone-on-bone pain that I had lived with day in, day out for years. From there, I continued to gain strength and felt much better physically. I was walking again and began to hike steeper and steeper paths. It was like regaining my freedom, and I am still feeling improvement and benefits more than seven months later. It has been an amazing experience."

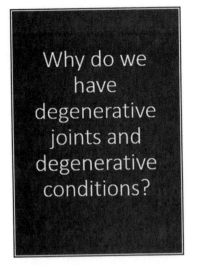

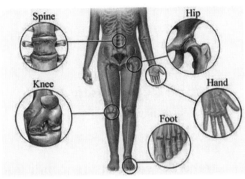

Your Body Is Degenerating with Age

Aging is a certainty; from this, there is no escape. But aging is a complex process and is different from person to person. Health and wellness is vastly different between people of the same age based on several factors.

The older we get, the more our bodies degenerate. It is well understood that muscle, bone, cartilage, and other body systems become less able, as we age, to repair themselves. That is why ailments tend to compound upon us the older we get.

Rarely do I see a patient who has only one issue, and the older they get, the more issues arise. Even stem cells are much more abundant at a younger age. The trouble is, we are trying to fix our health problems with patches that can make the problem worse. There are things we are putting in our bodies that are speeding up its degeneration.

When some of the most commonly prescribed treatments for degeneration are found to actually cause it, it can be frustrating to know where to go from there.

Top factors that cause or worsen degeneration:

- Cortisone injections
- Smoking
- Diet
- Obesity
- High blood pressure
- Alcohol
- Sugar

And other contributing conditions:

- Injury or trauma
- Genetic disorders
- Disease

There are other medical issues as well, problems with inflammation and certain medications, which can also worsen the degeneration.

As well, brain and physical health go hand in hand. We will investigate some studies that show a direct correlation between physical degeneration and mental impairment in a little while. Suffice it to say, regardless of where the inflammation starts, it spreads throughout the body. Patients struggle with few options on how to see more permanent improvement.

So, what has been done about degenerative conditions in the past? Or even currently? We have already mentioned cortisone injections, which are probably the most common (and arguably, the most destructive) option. In exchange for the weeks to months of respite from joint pain and inflammation that the injection provides, you get further degeneration and the opposite of healing.

People who have degenerative issues usually go through the same medical process:

Step 1: Physical therapy

A therapist will provide a list of exercises and activities to practice and some to avoid in order to allow for maximum healing of the affected area. Physical therapy works for some level of pain relief and encourages the body's natural healing tendencies.

Step 2: Prescription medication (painkillers)

Medication can relieve pain, but it also numbs the problem area, making it easy to reinjure it or prevent healing with too much activity. Other medications are prescribed to address specific aspects of various conditions, but they do not provide a cure.

Step 3: Cortisone injections

Cortisone injections are steroids injected into the problem area. This serves to reduce inflammation and usually improves chronic pain, but only temporarily. The real problem is that the cortisone injections actually cause degeneration, making the problem much worse over time.

Step 4: Surgery

Depending on the condition, surgery can either be a relatively simple day surgery or something like a heart transplant that requires many hours of surgery and weeks or months of recovery. Regardless of how serious the surgery is, there is always the potential for complications.

Step 5: Repeat

This often becomes a cycle, as there is no real reduction in inflammation or joint deterioration. It is much more destructive than it needs to be as well. People are not willing to stop and assess their issues; instead, they jump in, guns blazing.

With cortisone injections, they react immediately, reducing inflammation at the site of injection. Although it is an anti-inflammatory procedure, it does not last and ends up causing more harm than good. Some people react strongly to the cortisone and have severe degeneration as a result. As well, cortisone does not rebuild cartilage or tissue. In fact, it does the opposite.

Of all treatments, I would say cortisone injections are the most detrimental. Doctors continue to offer cortisone as a solution, often repeating injections three, four, or five times when the previous improvements disappear. Meanwhile, the so-called cure is actually breaking down the tissue and cartilage, making everything much worse.

Your body is already degenerating, so why speed up the process? Ultimately, when the injections stop working and the patient is desperate for another solution, knee replacement surgery or another more severe option is considered.

As far as knee replacements go, some people have great success with this surgery. Everything works the way it is supposed to; the patient is healed and never has any knee problems again.

At the same time, around 30 percent of patients who get knee replacements continue to have pain and inflammation in their repaired knees. Surgery does not address chronic inflammation, autoimmune disorders, or other issues that are affecting the knee.

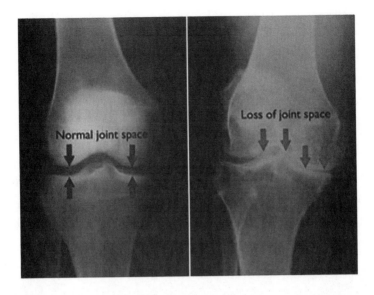

When not all the underlying health issues are addressed, more severe problems can occur. One recent study by the University of Florida, makes the correlation between knee replacement and cognitive decline.[2]

Published in the *Journal of Alzheimer's Disease*, the study discusses cases of people over the age of sixty who were having their knees replaced. One in four showed a decline in brain function after the surgery. And one in seven experienced decline across the entire brain system. Although they are not certain of the potential reason for this connection, it is believed to be related to inflammation in the brain.

When 25 percent of patients are experiencing mental function problems after a specific surgery, it gives one pause for thought. Is it a risk these patients are being told about before they agree to the surgery? I hope so.

---

[2]   http://www.ortho.ufl.edu/news/2018/03/09/one-five-older-adults-experience-brain-network-weakening-following-knee-replacement

This study and other studies of the same nature show how the connection between body systems is so much more intricate than we ever thought possible. What we will see from this is that stem cells, by their very nature, contribute to the healing processes of the entire body. It is what they are designed to do.

What Are Stem Cells and What Do They Do?

Stem cells are the body's original cells. From them, many other cells can grow. The Mayo Clinic describes the process by which stem cells divide to form more cells called *daughter cells*.[3] Daughter cells become either new stem cells or specialized cells that serve a specific function.

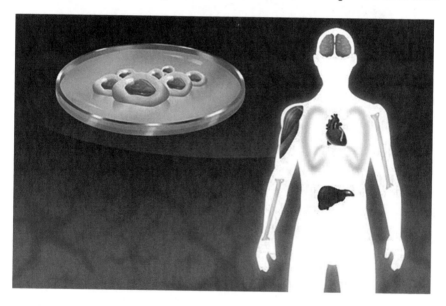

Stem cells are generated either naturally in the body or in a laboratory and are the only type of cell in the body that can regenerate into different cell types.

---

3   Mayo Clinic. *What are stem cells?* https://www.mayoclinic.org/tests-procedures/bone-marrow-transplant/in-depth/stem-cells/art-20048117

"This process of self-renewal and regeneration has long been seen as a potential fountain of youth and opportunity for whole-health healing."

The potential impact of having an abundance of cells specialized for regrowth is only beginning to be understood. As well, the list of potential areas of health improvement are endless. Some of the areas in which stem cells can become specialized are the following:

- Blood cells
- Brain cells
- Heart
- Muscle
- Bone and cartilage
- Skin and tissue
- Nerve cells

Stem cell therapy is a *nonsurgical way* of introducing regenerating cells to an area of ill-health. My colleagues and I have seen and heard from so many people who experienced substantial reduction in the chronic inflammation and pain that they had lived with for years.

This process has been used for years in multiple areas and industries, but it is taking time becoming common knowledge and accepted. That is mostly due to a lack of information. Athletes have used stem cell therapy for years, and it seems to be the direction that health care is headed.

Recently, changes in policy and regulation have made stem cell therapy much more attainable and at a more affordable cost for many. The important thing is that people now have the opportunity to hear about it, to learn what stem cell therapy is and how others have experienced it, giving everyone the option to find what is right for them.

I will go into an in-depth description of the different types of stem cell procedures and what they do in the next chapter. For now, suffice it to say that when people talk about stem cells, they are referring to *mesenchymal* stem cells (MSCs).

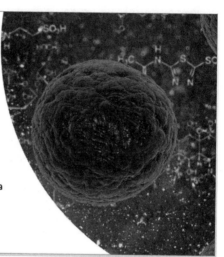

What are (Mesenchymal) Stem Cells?

- Regenerative cells of the body
- You all have them
- Live on your blood vessels and tissues
- Trauma, injury, cell aging /death trigger activation of stem cells via inflammation
- Inflammation attracts stem cells to the area needing repair and regeneration

Mesenchymal Stem Cells: Specialized cells that receive messages from other cells in the body and seek them out to provide regeneration and repair to the affected tissue.

Research has shown, in countless clinical studies and patient testimonials, that stem cells help repair muscle, bone, and tendons, leading to an overall stronger and healthier body. The reason the mesenchymal stem cells are so important is that they are part of our bodies already and designed to regenerate all our bodies' cells. As we get older, we have less and less of them, and so our bodies struggle and begin to degenerate.

Our natural stem cells reside in our blood and tissue, and they begin to die off during trauma, injury, or simply old age. Reinfusing your body with stem cells is a way to boost your systems, especially in the very specific regions you are having problems.

Sal's Story

"I have had chronic back pain for going on two decades. Depending on which doctor I saw, I got a different diagnosis, usually more than one. Arthritis was part of the problem, I knew that, but something else was going on.

"During the first decade, I was spending time trying to find some relief. I had been forced into early retirement because I couldn't physically do my job anymore. So there I was living day-to-day, miserable, and mostly stuck in the house. I couldn't get comfortable, I couldn't lie down, and I couldn't sleep. It was a nightmare.

"The pain is something that I will vividly remember all the days of my life. It was constant, and it went from dull to sharp and beyond. During all that time, I had chiropractic care and other treatments, and nothing made any difference.

"In my professional life, it was killing me. I spent a lot of my time alone because I was miserable. But I didn't want to have back surgery. Too many horror stories of failed back surgery and, I guess, my stubbornness to figure out what was going on brought me to look for alternative options.

"After having stem cell therapy, I feel so much better. I've got my life back, and I am able to find comfort. As soon as I got home from the experience, I slept well for the first time in years. Regaining my ability to sleep was huge, but it didn't end there. Slowly my overall health started to improve.

"For so many years, I was in pain and I did not know there was this option. And now, I feel like me, like I was given a fresh start *and a new lease on life. I am so thankful I overcame my hesitation and opened myself up to this new technique. The science behind it made sense, and I have met so many people whose lives have totally changed."*

Degeneration and Regeneration

Stem cells are attracted to areas of inflammation or those in need of repair and regeneration. Why, then, are people suffering from joint trouble and degenerative conditions, if the stem cells are supposed to be repairing these issues?

The answer involves an understanding of the balance of degeneration and regeneration and what that means to your health.

Degeneration: The loss of function in the cells of a tissue or organ primarily caused by inflammation

Regeneration: The ongoing rebuilding of tissues in the body

Both degeneration and regeneration are ongoing throughout our lives. Each one of them is a natural part of the body's processes. And they are both beneficial to some degree. In the same way inflammation is a natural part of the healing process, if it remains unchecked, it can cause disease.

When inflammation gets out of control, fatal diseases in many different areas such as those listed below are often the result:

- Pulmonary disease like COPD
- Cardiovascular disease
- Alzheimer's

- Diabetes
- Arthritis
- Autoimmune diseases

When inflammation is out of control, the degeneration and regeneration of cells is out of balance. Finding the cause of the inflammation will help provide an understanding of where the degeneration is. An increase in levels of stress and strain on the body is a major player in the degeneration of certain symptoms. Diet, sleep schedule, and lifestyle also impact the degeneration and regeneration processes.

These are the usually the aspects of our health that we can control. If you have a condition caused by degeneration in any area, ask yourself these questions to see if you can modify your lifestyle and see some improvement:

1. Am I getting adequate sleep so I feel rested when I wake up?
2. Do I stay up too late or wake frequently?
3. Is there any emotional stress from other people impacting my life?
4. How are my relationships with family, friends, or work colleagues?
5. Am I aware of any toxins in my environment?
6. What are my physical activity levels throughout each day?

By asking these questions, you can get a better picture of where and why degeneration is happening in your body and how you can encourage regeneration. All these questions are related to inflammation and cellular function. When there is *stress in the body*, or we are bombarded by medications, the natural process of regeneration cannot keep up with the rapid degeneration that is occurring.

Another difficulty our bodies have in regeneration is the reduction in number of stem cells over time. Since they are the main repair mechanism in our bodies and are anti-inflammatory super cells, they have a big job. The trouble is that the amount of stem cells we have decreases as we age.

When we are born, we have a high number of stem cells and very little need to use them. As time goes on, the stem cells become overloaded and eventually die. It is part of aging, and our bodies do not have the ability to keep up indefinitely.

The Age Factor

Getting older is inevitable and an undeniable experience everyone will have. During the aging process, degeneration of the body's functions occurs on a cellular level. As this happens, the inflammatory process of degeneration overwhelms the system's ability to fight it off.

Still, there are forces at play that we are only beginning to understand. People do not all age in the same way or at the same speed. We all get older, but people of the same age are in physiologically very different stages. Have a look, if you can, on your social media feed at a group of people you knew decades ago, or in high school. Some of them have hardly changed at all, and others are unrecognizable.

When degeneration begins, it accelerates the aging process, as the body struggles to keep up. At the same time, we do not regenerate as fast as we used to. So, what makes some of us better able to optimally repair and regenerate our bodies' systems? Here are some of the factors that affect the aging process:

- Physical injury or trauma
- Disease
- Stress level and management
- Genetic predisposition

Age is a factor for all major conditions. When people are facing major surgery, a knee or hip replacement, their bodies are degenerating at a much faster rate. At the same time, they are slower to regenerate, and their healing and recovery time, therefore, will be increased. The less invasive the process, the easier it is to integrate into the system.

Amy - Avoided Knee Surgery and Improved Outlook on Life

At 70 years old, I had been having knee pain for half my life. When I had my meniscus repaired, it felt better briefly and then it got bad right away. Worse than it had ever been before.

I could not perform normal daily activity and in the last year, it became sedentary because of pain. My life was closing in on me and I was becoming depressed thinking about the downward spiral and what would become of me.

Eventually, I resigned myself to surgery as my last chance. Then one night I stumbled upon one of Dr. Banerjee's videos about his stem cell therapy and healing program and it was like a light went on.

As a retired nurse, I had heard about stem cells years and years ago. Since they had been studying it for a long time, I thought long term results must be available and it was worth a shot.

Instead of major surgery with a possibly difficult outcome, I got stem cell therapy instead. Then, within 24 hours my knee pain disappeared.

In the first week I noticed other health issues seemed to vanish into thin air:

1. The neck and shoulder pain no longer kept me up at night.
2. My shortness of breath and rapid heartbeat disappeared.
3. I had normal blood pressure; no more medicine required.
4. I had improved energy and overall wellness.

Now I recommend stem cell therapy to anyone. It is the wave of the future in my opinion, from my medical background and the research that has been done. Anyone suffering pain from injury, lack of energy or other chronic problems needs to give it a try.

I am sleeping so much better now and without pain. I no longer look at the future in doom but now I know I will experience a lot of exciting new adventures.

The Remarkable Potential of Stem Cells

Autoimmune issues, chronic pain conditions, and inflamed joints are all degenerative situations that worsen with age. None of them have a cure or treatment that provides long-term solutions without invasive action and serious risk.

What can stem cells do?

- Reduce inflammation
- Balance the immune system
- Regenerate cell function
- Repair systems
- Revitalize old stem cells

Some critics of stem cell therapy cite patients who have seen no improvement, and these cases do happen. In the next chapter, we will go into this a little bit more, but the type of stem cells used in the therapy make all the difference to how effective it will be.

There are two main forms of stem cell therapies offered:

- **Autologous:** Stem cells are taken from the patient's own body.
- **Allogeneic:** Stem cells are received from a donor.

When stem cells come from the patient's own body (bone marrow or fat), a surgical procedure is required. Thus, there is an increase in pain and healing time. As you get older, you have fewer stem cells anyway. Studies show a correlation between autoimmune disorders and a decline in stem cells.

This option is more expensive and is seen to be less effective. On the other hand, when stem cells come from a donor, they can have more immediate results. The regenerative tissues are rejuvenated, and there is a burst of stem cells into the blood, providing response in the locations needed.

When stem cells are injected into the body, they seek out inflammation and provide repair. As well, depending on where they are used, they can revitalize different systems throughout the body.

The first patient I saw had stem cell therapy done on both knees. One of them was hurt in an injury twenty years ago and had never been the same since. He walked with a permanent limp and had to give up skiing, his passion. He received stem cells in each knee and noticed an immediate reduction in pain. He is now very active, skiing regularly, and has not used a cane since.

The way he put it was that it felt like the stem cell therapy was accelerating the healing processes in his body. And by knowing how the process works and what stem cells do, you can see that makes a lot of sense. We have yet to uncover and document the true breadth of potential for what stem cell therapy can do.

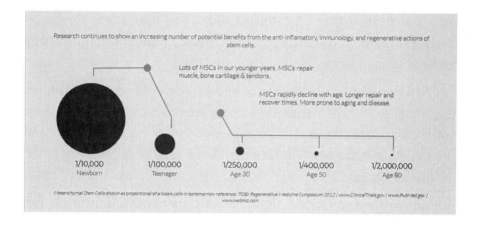

Research continues to show an increasing number of potential benefits from the anti-inflamatory, immunology, and regenerative actions of stem cells.

Lots of MSCs in our younger years. MSCs repair muscle, bone cartilage & tendons.

MSCs rapidly decline with age. Longer repair and recover times. More prone to aging and disease.

| 1/10,000 | 1/100,000 | 1/250,000 | 1/400,000 | 1/2,000,000 |
| Newborn | Teenager | Age 30 | Age 50 | Age 80 |

Mesenchymal Stem Cells shown as proportional of a totals cells in bonemarrow reference: TOBI Regenerative Medicine Symposium 2012 | www.ClinicalTrials.gov | www.PubMed.gov | www.webmd.com

Benefits of Regenerative Medicine

If you are looking to improve the quality of your life, reduce or eliminate pain, and get back to enjoying a healthy lifestyle, then stem cell therapy is a regenerative medical therapy that is safe and affordable.

Regenerative medicine is the science of living cells being used to potentially regenerate or facilitate the repair of cells damaged by disease, genetics, injury, or simple aging by stimulating the body's own repair mechanisms.[4] Research continues to ensure safe, ethical, and regulated processes are available to study the benefits of stem cell therapy and regeneration for healing.

---

[4]   Regen Medicine. *What is regenerative medicine?* http://regenmedicine.com/

CHAPTER 2

The History of Stem Cells

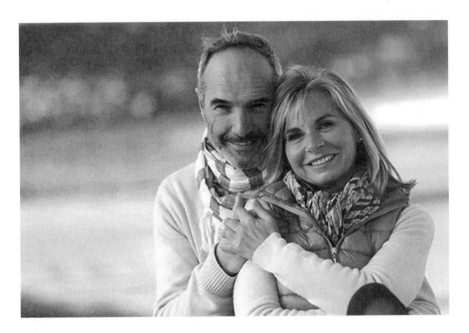

Where Transformation Begins

The healing revolution has begun as people are no longer willing to stand idly by while their bodies degenerate. People are waking up to the possibility of new options for problems that have been hampering their lives for years.

That is where it begins. Transforming lives and using cells for medicine is changing the history of the medical system as it shines light on a new path.

The healing properties of our bodies can be used and rejuvenated. It is a matter of science and learning from those who came before us. Our bodies really do have the ability to heal themselves, given the right treatment plan.

Following the advances in regenerative medicine, we can give our healing process assistance through stem cell therapy. Using techniques developed and improved upon over time provides safe and effective benefits for patients with different conditions.

When patients comes to my clinic to begin their journey toward health, they are looking for a game changer. Offering a cutting-edge therapy is as simple as following the science. Proper procedures and regulations are built into the systems behind the science.

Stem cells are a part of the body's natural repair kit. The history of the early use of stem cells compared to how we are using them now shows just how far we have come in our understanding of regeneration and degeneration.

Moving toward a health-care system that favors whole-health healing, the advancement of science is shedding light on the wide range of uses for stem cells in patients with many different conditions. Human studies are being undertaken to broaden the boundaries and potential conditions that can experience benefits from stem cell therapy.

While research continues, stem cell therapy is being offered in medical practices at a growing rate, as patients are seeking healing alternatives. As patients take matters into their own hands, they are finding out exactly what stem cell therapy has to offer.

The types of patients using stem cell therapy include those with the following conditions:

- Chronic pain
- Autoimmune issues

- Crohn's
- MS (multiple sclerosis)
- Spinal cord injury
- Joint or bone problems
- Skin damage and other wounds
- Arthritis
- Diabetes
- Parkinson's People are finding relief and hope in regenerative medicine. With the anti-inflammatory and healing properties of stem cells, they are seeing improvements without undergoing a serious procedure or surgery.

The field is evolving and expanding daily as the focus shifts to more specific applications. As always, the focus is on finding a method that enhances your own body's natural healing properties in order to achieve a better quality of life.

Bob's Story—Needed Knee Replacement

"My name is Bob, and I am recovering from chronic pain. I can also be a bit sarcastic and have been told I make a bit of a tough patient. And I will be the first to admit it. The worse my condition got, the more frustrated I became. Face it, I was pissed off. My whole life, I mastered my body; I played college ball and kept active in multiple sports as an adult. That was until my knees started to give out.

"It was my right knee that was the biggest mess. Watching me get out of a chair was darn near unsightly as I groaned, my bones cracking against each other. The worse it got, the more

bitter I became. My knees meant my freedom, and I am not one to sit still.

"Everyone kept telling me that I am not getting any younger. Well, I thought (and still do) that was bull. I am rolling past seventy, but I have seen guys in their eighties playing golf like it's nothing.

"I knew it was more than just age, but no one was able to give me answers that led to any improvement. It was frustrating to say the least.

"The orthopedic surgeon said I would need a new knee in less than five years, but if I didn't take it easy, then it wouldn't last half that time. I was so tired of being told to take it easy. After going to physical therapy for half a year, it was time to try something new. The PT helped with the stiffness, but it was not doing anything to actually solve my day-to-day health problems.

"Enough was enough, and I became obsessed with finding something else to help me. I did not want to live my last years out like this at all. My right knee was much worse than my left, but then I began favoring it, and it was causing problems for the left knee.

"Deep down, a feeling of dread started to creep into being. As I started to feel worse and worse, it felt like a slow progression to death. So when I heard about stem cell therapy, I knew it was now or never.

"After I had the treatment, the stiffness and cracking reduced immediately. Four weeks later, and I was using the recumbent bike and just getting around so much better. It has been remarkable how I just continue to get better. And happy news for those

around me—everyone says I am much less grouchy and bitter. I can't help it. Even my sarcasm is reduced as I feel like I have a new lease on life.

"If I had to say one thing to anyone looking for more information, it is that stem cell therapy is the one option I found with the least possible risks or side effects. Do yourself a favor and look into it. You really have nothing to lose. And if you are like me, you might have the benefit of regaining a significant portion of your health."

The History of Stem Cells

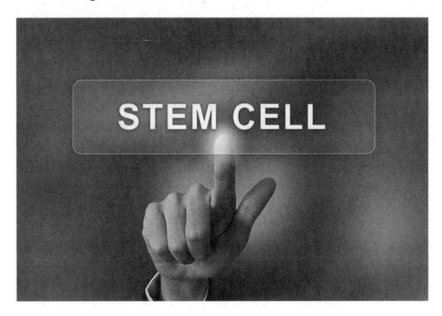

Stem cell therapy is only recently becoming a hot topic in the health and wellness field, even though it has been around for decades. The research on stem cells started in the 1900s, when it was discovered that some cells were able to create new blood cells.

Stem cell therapy has come a long way since then, as the science and public opinion have offered varied opinions on the effectiveness and ethics of the procedure. A timeline of more than a century of research, policy, and clinical trial shows how far we have come:[4]

1909: Alexander Maximow described the theory that all blood cells originate from the same cell.

1936: Blood transfusions, done as early as World War I, are a form of stem cell therapy.

1968: First successful bone-marrow transplant to treat extremely deficient immune systems in two siblings.

1972: Umbilical cord blood used to treat leukemia.

1978: First stem cells developed from mice. In the same year, stem cells were discovered in human cord blood.

1981: In vitro stem cell line first developed from mice.

1988: First stem cells developed from a primate. As well, embryonic stem cell lines were developed from a hamster.

1990: First cord blood transplant in a nonrelated patient.[4]

1995: Research into stem cells and autoimmune disorders. The first embryonic stem cell line from a primate was created.

1997: A lamb was cloned using stem cells. The same year a leukemia connection to hematopoietic stem cell was found. Dolly, the sheep, was created at the Roslin Institute in Edinburgh, when scientist fused a sheep egg with an udder cell and implanted it in a surrogate mother sheep.

1997–2004: Several cord blood banks are developed.

1998: First stem cells developed from a human.

1999–2000: Scientists discovered stem cells could be obtained from different tissue and bone marrow in mice.

2001: President George W. Bush limits U.S. federal funding on stem cell research.

2005: A university in South Korea makes fraudulent claims about successful cloning using human stem cells. At the same time, improvements are made in the efficiency of cord blood transplants. As well, research is being done in regard to the response to stem cell therapy in patients with a spinal cord injury.

2006: Kyoto University in Japan discovered a process to reprogram adult stem cells to make them embryonic-like cells.

2007: Three scientists receive the Nobel Prize for their stem cell research on genetics and embryonic stem cells. Dr. Anthony Atala completed research that showed a new type of stem cell had been isolated in amniotic fluid.

2009: President Barack Obama revokes U.S. funding limits on stem cell research.

2010: A patient with a spinal cord injury receives the first medical treatment of stem cells in Menlo Park, California. In the same year, a stem cell therapy to treat blindness was studied with positive results.

2012: Another scientist wins a Nobel Prize for work on stem cells. As well, a clinical trial at John Hopkins University resulted in the successful regrowth of new heart tissue after a patient who had had a heart attack received stem cell therapy.

2013: U.S. Supreme Court declined to hear a major case that would have prevented further stem cell research. The decision was seen as a step in the right direction for ethical research. A study of stem cell therapy for diabetics was also completed with favorable results.

2014: Trials begin on stem cell therapy to improve conditions that cause blindness.

2016: President Obama signs the 21st Century Cures Act into law, allowing for adequate response time in regenerative medicine research results. It is anticipated that this will streamline the procedures and requirements for alternative-healing options such as stem cell therapy.

2017: Study of umbilical cord stem cells for patients with arthritis.

Since stem cells were discovered, there has been the release of controversial, unethical, and fraudulent information and resources regarding the science of the therapies. It is important not to let these inaccuracies get in the way of the science behind what is happening.

The history of stem cells sheds light on how it has been received by the medical community and beyond to the average patient. As science continues to build on the research and work that has been done over the past few decades, new breakthroughs are expected.

How Stem Cells Were First Used

In the early 1990s, stem cells began to be used through bone-marrow transplants to treat multiple diseases and conditions. A little more than a decade later, research determined that stem cells could prevent rejection in organ-transplant patients.[4]

This process sought to change the reaction of the body to the transplant. So that instead of treating the transplant as a foreign body to attack, through the help of the stem cells, the recipient's immune system would accept the transplant and begin to heal.

Although this test was done in the laboratory with rats, it could soon be replicated in human trials. Scientists expect that, eventually, stem cell therapy could be used in conjunction with organ transplants and would negate the need for immune-suppressant drugs.

Regenerative medicine started out on the fringe of the industry. Now that more is known about these applications and how they are connected to whole-body health, stem cell therapy is becoming accepted on a much-wider scale.

Over time, more clinical studies and research have taken place to the extent that stem cells are fast becoming more common for a multitude of ailments. Since the 1970s, advances in the production of umbilical cord stem cells has made the therapy available to a wider group of people.

Ongoing clinical studies are showing positive outcomes with stem cells involved in the following ailments:

- Spinal cord injury
- Cerebral palsy
- Encephalopathy
- Diabetes
- Heart disorders
- Neurological disorders
- Autoimmune conditions

Moving forward, with people seeking relief from pain caused by all kinds of disorders, this new movement in medicine will become more mainstream. As long as advancements continue to be supported by people and policy, science and research will continue to find new hope in the health care.

Mary's Story—Terrible Ankle Clicking

"I first heard of stem cells, years ago, when a cousin had a transplant. Apparently, they used stem cells as part of the procedure, and another relative was going on and on about what a horrible treatment it was. Of course, I didn't know it at the time, but stem cell therapy would one day change my life.

"For as long as I can remember, all of my adult life, I had a clicking in my ankle, and it was, what I considered weak. It didn't affect me too much, at first, though as I got older, I developed arthritis,

which seemed to make the whole situation a lot more difficult to deal with and much more painful.

"It became too unbearable to walk. I used crutches if I had to move, but remained immobile in discomfort for the most part. My work was being affected, and instead of enjoying my last year before retirement, I dreaded trying to keep up with my duties and mask my pain.

"All along, I had been prescribed painkillers, though I tried not to take them unless I needed them. A close friend had confided that her divorce had been caused by an addiction to painkillers, and she did not want to see me go down that road. And I agreed with her. For the most part, I saved the pills for when I was really bad, especially at night.

"When I moved at night, the pain kept me awake for hours. Since I tend to move around in my sleep a lot, I was awake a lot. Then the lack of sleep started adding new symptoms, and it was all becoming so overwhelming.

"During the days I did go out, I was tired of being treated differently because of my crutches. My day-to-day life was consumed with trying to figure out how I would get it all done.

"When I heard about the stem cell therapy I knew it was for me, right away, although the initial questions and prep felt daunting to my unfamiliar self. Less than three days later, I was off my crutches. Right away, I noticed the pain was much less, and I was amazed.

"Everyone around me noticed the biggest changes before me. They said they could not believe how much less tense I was. As well,

I was getting out more and had a much more cheerful overall attitude on life.

"You really don't realize how much the pain is wearing you down. How chronic pain really is debilitating, and you start to lose yourself. After therapy, it was like a weight had been lifted, and I could be me again. What a wonderful feeling."

Two Types of Stem Cell Therapies

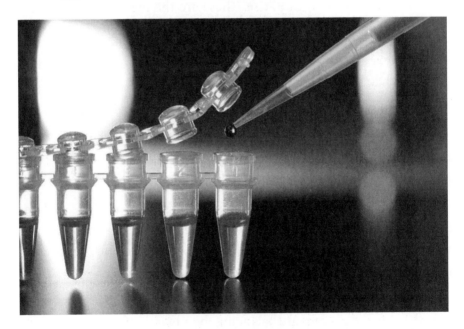

We will go into the science of stem cell therapy in the next chapter. No need to overwhelm you with all the details at once. Instead, let's take it bit by bit, based on how stem cells work together with your body's systems to repair and regenerate, and to improve health and well-being.

In the previous chapter, we defined the two types of stem cell therapies:

- **Autologous:** Harvested from your own body and then processed to be used in stem cell therapy for your specific ailment.
- **Allogeneic:** There are two types of allogeneic, (1) the amniotic/placenta (this is **not** what we use), and (2) the umbilical cord stem cells taken from cord blood after childbirth, under specific regulations.

The biggest challenge using autologous stem cells is the surgical requirements. When the stem cells are taken from you, there is pain and complications that can arise. These are the most common places from which stem cells are taken:

- Bone marrow
- Pelvic bone
- Fat

Basically, autologous stem cell therapy is adding a medical process to an already fragile system. Recovery time is increased, and the body has to work twice as hard to prevent infection and regain health.

Another consideration is that the patient's stem cells are as old as the patient. So if you are over forty and already have health issues, you will be drawing from an empty well, so to speak. The older we get, the lower the quality and quantity of our stem cells become.

People who seek out stem cell therapy obviously have issues with how their own stem cells are balancing their health. If you already have chronic inflammation, pain, and joint problems, this type of therapy might not be as successful for you.

As well, autologous therapy is the most expensive form of stem cell therapy, because it requires a much-more involved process.

Allogeneic stem cell therapy avoids all that extra trauma by getting stem cells from healthy donors. No surgical procedure is required, which makes the process much simpler.

Using donor cells offers multiple benefits:

- Health of cells is predetermined
- Testing is done for safety and viability
- Easy and simple procedure, without fatal risk
- 100 percent ethically sourced stem cells
- Stem cells are very young in age and have not yet begun to degenerate
- All the factors in the procedure are easy to anticipate and control
- Customized number of cells, specific to the individual needs
- Therapy can be done on more than one area at a time—more efficient
- Umbilical cord stem cells provide an unlimited supply of naturally occurring donor cells

Look at it from the perspective of a patient. Many patients struggle with knee problems. Usually, the pain has expanded enough that it has taken over some aspect of their lives. So then, if they undergo autologous therapy, it becomes a more complex surgical procedure with unclear quality, rather than a straightforward experience with a safe and effective product.

Of course, every patient is different, and everyone has different health considerations. But often, when stem cells are taken from patients for use on themselves, more than double the amount of cells is required. Depending on the patient's age, such a significant volume of stem cells removed from the bone marrow, or elsewhere, can take a while to heal.

As well, it is not as easy to know the efficacy of stem cells taken from an unwell patient. If there are signs that the patient's body is struggling to heal, stem cell therapy using autologous stem cells could actually be doing more harm than good.

On the other hand, with allogeneic stem cell therapy, there is a much higher success rate because the number and quality of stem cells is known beforehand. And since the procedure is nonsurgical, results are often seen much sooner.

That is why it is so easy to do multiple procedures in one with allogeneic stem cell therapy. Since we order the stem cells in the quantity required, it is quite simple to get exactly the amount we need for each patient.

Allogeneic stem cells are divided into three categories:

1. **Amniotic and Placental:** We do *not* use this allogeneic process in our practice, but some places do use amniotic fluid for their stem cell therapy. Amniotic fluid is not consistent, and there is potential to have miscellaneous debris.

    Stem cells from the placenta have a high concentration from the mother, so they are not the youngest or most effective option. As well, placental cells can cause an allergic or immune reaction, which can cause complications for the patient.

2. **Bone Marrow:** This is another process that we do not use in our clinic. Stem cells from bone marrow were some of the first used. Still, it can be invasive for the donor, and the age of the stem cells must be taken into consideration. This can cause conflict, and is unnecessary, when the third option is more efficient.

3. **Umbilical Cord Blood:** Stem cells are taken from the umbilical cord blood, after it has been separated from the mother and baby. This is 100 percent noninvasive and uses vital stem cells

that are often thrown away. With umbilical cord blood, the health of the donor is predetermined, and a number of other safety factors are easier to control.

Mesenchymal stem cells are the specialized cells that receive the distress calls from the other systems in your body. From there, stem cells seek out inflammation and work on regeneration. The younger the donor supply, the higher the concentration of mesenchymal stem cells within the sample.

Umbilical cord blood contains stem cells, growth factors, and immune cells that are immature as they have to be compatible to both mother and child, so are more adaptable in nature. In our clinic, the umbilical cord blood we use comes from Regen Medicine, who provide safe and effective, FDA-compliant stem cells.

The Quality of Stem Cells We Use

Here is the reason why we use the stem cells that we do in our therapies: so we can do everything in our power to offer the safest and highest-quality option. Umbilical cord stem cells are the youngest potential source that actively replicate throughout the body very quickly.

Since they are at peak efficiency, stem cells from the umbilical cord double every twenty-four to twenty-eight hours. By the time we are forty years old, it takes forty hours, and at the age of sixty-five, our stem cells take sixty hours. The faster the cells divide, the more beneficial they are on the healing properties of the body.

The stem cells we use are chosen to prevent some of the issues that occur with other stem cell therapies—for example:

- Potential for allergic reaction
- Low quantity of stem cells based on age or illness

- Complications from a surgical procedure like bone marrow harvesting, or getting the fat cells out of a live donor
- Reduced efficiency of older stem cells over time
- Improper screening of stem cells prior to therapy

So, what happens when these stem cells are injected into the patient? Imagine, if you will, just one of the stem cells and watch it regenerate. In thirty days, one umbilical cord stem cell would grow to more than one billion. If that same stem cell came from an adult, forty years old, it would become 32,000 cells. And if it were a stem cell from a sixty-five-year old, that same cell would grow into only 200 stem cells.

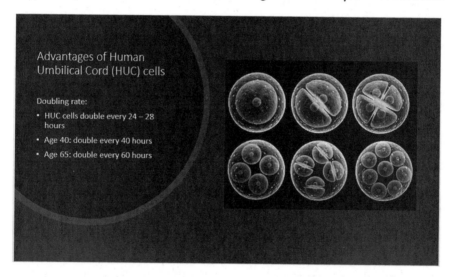

This makes a very vivid picture showing how and why umbilical cord stem cells work in the best interest of the patient's health. This stem cell therapy usually results in much-more significant changes, more quickly, and over a longer duration of time. When stem cells are put into the body, they last sixty-five cycles before they are pushed back out.

While regenerating, they release anti-inflammatory factors, as well as immune system and growth factors. Using stem cells from the umbilical cord gives continued benefits due to the nature of these young cells.

Some people voice concerns about the donor stem cells becoming part of their new tissue. However, this is not really what happens. When cells are put into the body, regardless of whether they are from the patient or a donor, they do not become part of your body's tissue. Instead, they help the body repair its own tissue and regenerate.

The benefits of umbilical cord stem cells are being continuously researched with some interesting findings being discovered:

- A study by the University of Paris showed improvement can last up to eighteen years after only one experience
- The youngest stem cells are the most potent
- The more stem cells multiply, the more effective they are
- Of all therapy options, umbilical cord stem cells are nonallergenic

As research continues, the science points the way to this form of stem cell therapy. Of everyone with whom I have spoken who had stem cell therapy and yet saw no results, I asked the same question: "What type of stem cell therapy did you have done?" Every single person advised they had had autologous stem cell therapy.

For the most part, when people do not have success with stem cell therapy, it is because they used their own stem cells. Unfortunately, most of the patients are fifty, sixty, seventy, or eighty years old, and so they have fewer stem cells to begin with. Then they are subjected to an intense process of surgery before the stem cell therapy, and the whole system becomes much less effective.

What we are beginning to realize is that, as stem cells get older, they secrete less anti-inflammatory factors and are not as readily able to encourage regeneration. The surprising outcome of this is that they can actually contribute damage to the already weakened area. On the other hand, umbilical cord stem cells actually help your older stem cells act younger.

Umbilical cord blood comes from the blood vessels of the umbilical cord after the baby has been delivered. At least three unique types of stem cells with different properties and features have been found in umbilical cord blood. There is yet to be a standardization of criteria for naming cord blood stem cells, so different terms have been used in different situations. Sometimes this can lead to misleading or inaccurate descriptions.

For the purposes of this book, we will simply explain the process as it is used in stem cell therapy. Instead of complicating matters with a long explanation, we are going to focus on how it works. By providing simple and exact descriptions, a clearer, more precise understanding becomes evident.

In our stem cell therapy procedure, a heterogeneous population of cells is used. This includes the three distinct categories found in umbilical cord blood:

1. **Hematopoietic Stem Cells:**
   Blood cells are formed through a process called hematopoiesis. It is an ongoing cycle of replenishment as new cells continually regenerate, divide, and differentiate.

2. **Mesenchymal Stem Cells:**
   This type of stem cell has found to be extremely versatile. Mesenchymal stem cells are able to regenerate into any other type of cell with ease. These cells are highly successful in stem cell therapy. Yet they are also found in the least quantity.

3. **Endothelial Stem Cells:**
   Found in connection to the vascular system, these stem cells are also able to differentiate for specialized systems. Endothelial stem cells also produce progenitor cells, which are less potent than their parent cell.

These stem cells work synergistically to complete their overall function. Each one supports different building blocks of life and promotes healing and regeneration in specific locations. Hematopoietic cells include erythrocytes and leukocytes.

Mesenchymal stem cells, which are similar to the ones found in bone marrow, receive signals from the body and help encourage functions of regeneration. Working together as the earliest foundations of growth, umbilical cord stem cells are showing remarkable ability in a wide variety of areas.

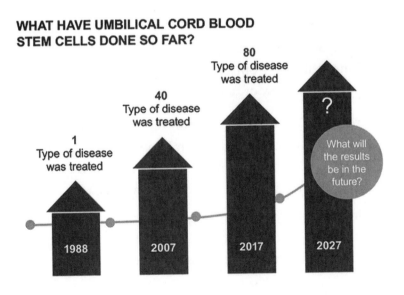

WHAT HAVE UMBILICAL CORD BLOOD STEM CELLS DONE SO FAR?

80
Type of disease was treated

40
Type of disease was treated

1
Type of disease was treated

?

What will the results be in the future?

1988   2007   2017   2027

Why Human Umbilical Cord Tissue?

There has been a lot of debate and controversy around stem cell therapy, especially considering rapidly advancing research and clinical applications. Every option has benefits and disadvantages.

Our reason for choosing human umbilical cord tissue is based on the scientific studies, experience, and feedback of clients. Having a safe and consistent supply of abundant stem cells provides the ability to offer dependable treatment tailored to the needs of the patient.

The resulting conclusion is the human umbilical cord tissue stem cells are the best option for successful results in our patients. If we can give our patients an optimal start to their healing journey, their chances of improvement increase. Umbilical cord stem cells provide this optimal situation in a variety of ways:

- Consistent quality and quantity of stem cells
- Safe and ethical retrieval of stem cells without the need of a live donor
- Abundance of all three types of stem cells within the cord blood
- Using stem cells from a supply that is often simply thrown away
- Unlimited supply of stem cells

According to World Health Organization statistics for 2011, the global birth rate has exceeded 140 million per year. This number highlights the availability of umbilical cord stem cells in a way that does not raise any ethical or controversial concerns.

Keeping up with the cutting edge of research and technology, we find that umbilical cord stem cells provide the most benefit with the least potential problems for everyone involved.

Human Umbilical Cord	• What we use
	• From umbilical blood and tissue
	• No potential for allergic reaction
	• Youngest most vital adult stem cells

Jack's Story—Chronic Pain from an Injury

"I thought my active life was done. Over the years, I had the odd injury, but nothing that ever kept me down for too long. Then it seemed I hit sixty-five, and everything happened at once.

" My condition worsened so quickly that I went from running marathons to not being able to keep up with my two-year-old grandson. I was watching him grow from the sidelines, and it broke my heart every time I had to say, "Sorry, grandpa is not feeling well," or "Be careful, don't jump on grandpa."

"I never was given a straight answer when trying to heal my chronic pain. At first, it was one thing, then another. The only things they were sure of were that there were no easy answers. It was suggested to me that I would have to go to the chiropractor once a week to get relief.

"So I tried that for a while but it didn't seem to help. It was time-consuming and expensive, and I was usually wiped out for the day after every appointment. After a while, I stopped going, and the pain mounted.

"When I saw the ad for stem cell therapy on television one day, I was interested because it said some people were getting rid of their pain. And it was not a surgical procedure. It piqued my interest, but I assumed I couldn't afford it, and kept living in pain.

"Not long afterwards, I found out my daughter was remarrying. She and my grandchildren had it rough for a while, and things were finally coming together for her. Her future husband was a good man, and it sparked hope in me again.

"It was like I needed the hope to come from somewhere outside my condition. I was so tired of all the appointments and trial medications, all for nothing. Now that my daughter shared her good news, I secretly made a promise to myself to find a way to walk her down the aisle pain-free.

"It was my newfound determination to dance at her wedding. While chewing over my options, I came across stem cell therapy again and decided to give it a try. Although I had close to a year until my daughter's wedding, I was ready to dance months earlier.

"In fact, the initial results on my knee were so promising, I continued the process for the pain throughout my body. My shoulder, back, and hip were all part of a bigger inflammation problem going on inside me. And every time I used stem cell therapy, I saw improvement in one or more areas.

"Finally, I can breathe again without every part of my body tensed in pain. And life is no longer so dreary. Everything seems much more positive as I can get out and enjoy and experience different things. I even have the energy to watch my grandchildren once a week to give my daughter and her new husband some time together.

"Being able to sleep properly and walk without pain are not things people usually think about. When you have to think about them, though, they are earth-shatteringly important. Don't underestimate the power of whole-body healing."

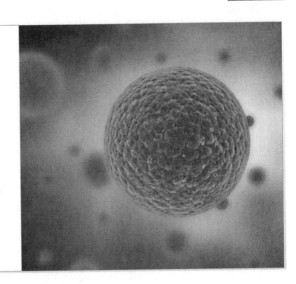

Is There Clinical Research?

A search of www.clinicaltrials.gov provides information on more than 5300 clinical trials being conducted worldwide

The Personal and the Practical Choice

Choosing stem cell therapy is a personal matter, as each individual has a different life experience and need. The practical aspect that everyone wants to know, before they go further, is what clinical research has been done.

Although it is a relatively new therapy, research is ongoing and expanding exponentially year after year. Scientific studies are sharing positive results, especially in autoimmune- or inflammation-related conditions. Many other conditions are being added to research trials every year, as regenerative medicine is looking to become the forefront of the future of health care.

Much of the research is and will be referenced in this book for easy access. As well, there are additional resources at *clinicaltrials.gov* or *PubMed*. These sites offer clinical research papers on the worldwide stem cell therapy progress.

These scientific trials are looking into the vast array of areas stem cell therapy can be used, including treatment for the following conditions:

- Muscles, joints, and tendons
- Chronic pain
- Autoimmune disorders
- Inflammation
- Cardiovascular issues
- Bone degeneration
- Nerve damage

As research continues, the future of stem cell therapy is advancing toward targeting specific tissues, organs, and conditions. At this point, *more than 5000 clinical trials* are ongoing or have been completed.

Another concern potential patients face is the possibility of side effects. Most people are used to receiving a long list of possible side effects from medical treatments and medications. However, there really are not any side effects from human umbilical cord stem cell therapy. One of the reasons why this option is so favorable is that there are no major complications associated with it.

The only minor occurrences could be a slight irritation at the site of the injection and sometimes flu-like symptoms for twenty-four to forty-eight hours. And actually, these are a good sign that there is a change occurring.

The most personal aspect of this whole process is the overall success of the stem cell therapy. In the end, every person will determine how successful it is based on their own experience and criteria.

The following is a list we use to gauge how well the therapy has benefited a patient:

- Reduction in pain level
- Improvement in mobility
- Ability to participate in hobbies and daily life
- Change in quality of life
- Increase in energy level
- Decreased swelling and inflammation
- Overall improvement in mood and well-being

All of these together give us a good indication as to how the stem cell therapy has assisted the patient in accomplishing personal health goals. From the time a patient enters the office, the process is streamlined for *the patient's* needs.

After an initial consultation, we look at all aspects of your condition and history. The problems you have and other factors involved will help you discover whether stem cell therapy might be a good option for you. From there, you will complete a medical appointment where the stem cell therapy occurs.

Six weeks later, we have a follow-up visit to review your progress. And again, twelve weeks after the stem cell treatment, we complete a final evaluation. This gives us a broad perspective of your continued health.

From the beginning, it is our intent to make sure everyone has the proper information. The history of the research and the science behind stem cell therapy is leading to promising new revelations. Following the science and the studies gives all parties the opportunity to understand stem cell therapy and see how it fits in their own health goals.

CHAPTER 3

The Science behind Stem Cells

Stem Cell Sources

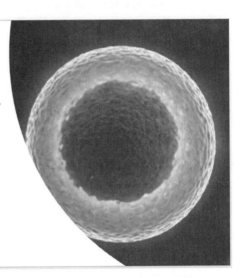

Stem Cell Therapy

- Direction healthcare is headed
- Used by athlete's for 10+ years
- Changes in rules & regulations have allowed stem cell therapy to be available at reasonable cost

Stem cell therapy is not going anywhere as people's experiences and results continue to speak for themselves. For this reason, the science and research involved must be maintained to ensure safety and efficacy.

Proper legislation, regulation, and oversight are being developed for each individual type of stem cell therapy. This is necessary as not all sources and procedures are carried out in the same way. As well, some sources that raise ethical concerns must not be lumped in with safe products from sustainable sources.

The main objections and controversial aspects of stem cell research should not be understated. There are ethical questions, and it is essential the proper procedures and oversight are in place. To simplify this process, stem cell therapies need to be divided into groups based on the source of the stem cells.

Stem Cell Source and Definition

1. **Adult stem cells:** Cells from mature bone marrow and fat tissue
2. **Donor stem cells:** Cells from someone other than the patient
3. **Embryonic stem cells:** Cells from human embryo
4. **Fetal stem cells:** Cells from aborted fetuses
5. **Placental stem cells:** Cells from placenta or amniotic fluid
6. **Umbilical cord blood stem cells:** Cells from the umbilical cord, after birth

There are some sources that might be more problematic than others. Once people differentiate among the sources and understand that our therapies use a source of safe and ethically obtained stem cells, they are usually ready to move on to improving their health.

From there, we begin to investigate the science of how stem cell therapy has helped others. Working and partnering with professionals, from the source of our stem cells to the follow up after the procedure, provides each patient with assurance of our level of care.

In our office, the main conditions my colleagues and I see are those associated with inflammation and joint pain including the following:

- Knees
- Shoulders
- Hips
- Ankles
- Neck

- Back
- Wrists
- Autoimmune issues
- Organ and intestinal function
- Other areas associated with arthritis

As part of a medical team, we collaborate, and my medical team and I look at each case study in my clinic together. As the educator and initial evaluator, I walk everyone through the process and then refer them to the rest of the medical team to complete the therapy.

Based on the symptoms of each patient, we might suggest stem cell therapy to improve these conditions:

- Chronic pain
- Mobility restrictions
- Autoimmune conditions
- Balance issues and vertigo
- Mental fog
- Energy level issues
- Hormonal balance

The other benefit we so often see, yet which is hard to name, is the altered outlook on life, the mood, and the peace that comes to patients. From finding the ideal source of stem cells to matching therapy with an individual patient's needs, we make their healing our top priority.

The science behind stem cells is part of every step we take as we work through solutions for our patients. Following the research papers from past and current studies and monitoring new advancements are part of our practice. As such, we partner with professionals and businesses that adhere to strict safety regulations. The future of stem cell therapy is broad, and by remaining aware of new advancements, we can fine-tune the therapies we offer our patients.

Potential Application of Human Stem Cells

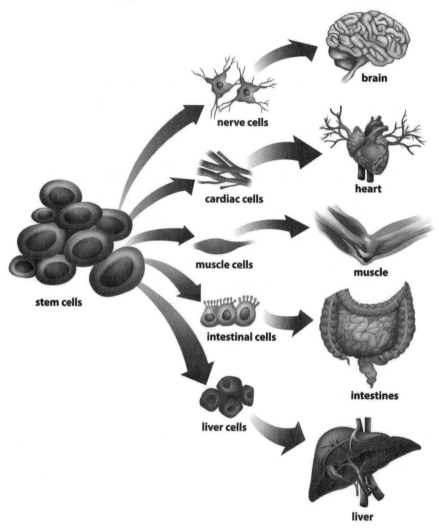

Yosef's Story—Autoimmune Condition

"I was diagnosed with an autoimmune condition, and I struggled for a long time to accept the diagnosis. I didn't want to hear it, and I wanted the doctor to be wrong. I told everyone who would listen why I thought the diagnosis was wrong.

"It wasn't the answer I was looking for, as I wanted to know what was wrong with me and how to fix it. I didn't want more tests and uncertainty; I have enough of that in my life as it is.

"Anyone who's been there with me knows that an autoimmune condition brings more questions than answers. And exhaustion—who had time to look for answers when I was constantly exhausted? I felt completely wiped out, no matter how long I slept.

"And I was so mad. I was just pissed off all the time; even when there was nothing bugging me, I was still so angry. I had just retired and planned a cruise to celebrate with my wife. We worked so hard for so many years; finally, I was retired, and we could go.

"Well of course, I was diagnosed two months before our trip, and I will admit, I was in rough shape. But when my doctor told me I couldn't travel, and my wife said it didn't matter because I couldn't get health insurance anyway, it was almost too much.

"It was our dream to travel, and it was all unravelling so fast. I could tell my wife was losing patience with my irritability and that I was always tired even though I slept so much. She tried to be patient, but there was a lot going on.

"Things were a bit tight financially, and my wife had wanted me to wait six months to retire. If I had listened to her, I would *have been off on sick leave with full pay and benefits, while accumulating more into our retirement fund.*

"As it was, I retired with something like 300 days of unused sick leave, so I could see why it bothered my wife. It got to me too, and it really messed with my head. I felt jinxed, like the universe was against me.

"I felt like my life was over, and at times, I wanted it to be. As time went on with no improvement, I went into a deep depression.

"My wife was at her wit's end, and I was lost. I was going to all these doctors, and nothing was working. And then, she found stem cell therapy. She told me to look into it and believed it would help me.

"Of course, I was skeptical, and probably a bit rude, on that first meeting. I was tired of the BS frankly and figured this doctor would be the same as the others, with no real valuable help to offer.

"What's more is that all my questions were being answered, and they made me feel at ease. There were videos and written materials detailing the science and research behind it. I really got the sense that they knew what they were doing, and even more important, they cared about my health.

"My wife comes with me to all of my appointments because I usually forget what they tell me. She said that was the first time she was acknowledged or recognized at any appointment. Usually, they just ignored her, but here she was part of the discussion because she saw how it was affecting my life.

"That was huge for me, and after going over everything again over a cup of tea with my wife, I decided to go for it. And it was amazing. The staff was all so friendly, kind, and genuine. I felt at ease the whole time, and I was a new person the very next day.

"Now I can smell again. Food tastes better, my bowels are working better, and just simply put, life feels better. Where before, I couldn't sleep on my left side, couldn't sleep comfortably much at all. At two or three in the afternoon, I was exhausted and just done for the day. It was awful.

"Now I am cleared to travel and finally replanning that cruise we have been waiting to take. Stem cell therapy was a game changer for me. It was a light at the end of a very dark tunnel."

Science and Research

As we saw in chapter 2, research on stem cells is not new. The science has been studied and treatments have been ongoing for decades with no foreseeable drawbacks. As research continues, new breakthroughs are being made frequently.

Now that laws are in place to protect and support stem cell research, it is expected that the research will exceed expectations, as the benefits of stem cells becomes widely accepted.

When stem cells were discovered, it was found that these groups of cells were the impetus for growth and regeneration throughout the body. When stem cells divide, they can become cells with a new function. In this way, our earliest cells develop from an embryo into a human with all the parts in the right place. Because of stem cells, our bodies develop cells for all the different parts of the whole body, including these:

- Skeletal system
- Nervous system
- Muscular system
- Cardiovascular system
- Immune system
- Circulatory system
- Digestive system
- Endocrine system
- And all the parts and processes that support these systems

Studies are being done on the effectiveness of stem cell therapy on over forty diseases, illnesses, and conditions. Many of these are degenerative in nature, which makes sense from a scientific perspective. Since stem cells provide regeneration and anti-inflammatory properties, new young cells can provide relief to systems that have been fighting illness for so long.

Knowing and understanding how stem cells work, including their regenerative properties, give a good understanding as to how stem cell therapy works in each individual case. Choosing stem cells that are versatile and easily adaptable to new requirements enables stem cell therapy to target a patient's condition and give the body a boost in regaining the pathway to health.

There are promising results showing benefits of stem cell therapy on degenerative conditions such as these:

- Lupus
- Crohn's
- Degenerative bone conditions
- Hip, knee, and shoulder pain
- Skin problems and wound healing

- Diabetes
- Parkinson's
- Alzheimer's
- Endometriosis
- Asthma
- COPD (chronic obstructive pulmonary disease)
- Thyroid disorders
- IBS (irritable bowel syndrome)

Patients see rapid improvements with stem cell therapy because the donor cells from the umbilical cords are dispersed right at the heart of the problem. From there, they can start working immediately to regenerate and reduce inflammation.

Public opinion is catching up with science and research as the results speak for themselves. As time goes on, safe and professional health-care providers are looking to increase the availability of stem cell therapy.

Predictive Biothech

Predictive Biotech provides human cell and tissue transplant products that contain cytokines, growth factors, hyaluronic acid, endothelial cells, epithelial cells and mesenchymal stromal cells; or mesenchymal stem cells as the clinical community and general public refer to them. They are a safe, effective, and affordable option for cutting-edge regenerative medicine.

Predictive Biotech's products are FDA-compliant and sourced from the rich Wharton's Jelly layer of the umbilical cord and amniotic fluid and amnio tissue from healthy, full-term donors. Predictive Biotech's products are meticulously handled every step of the way. Carefully collected from thoroughly screened, full-term birth tissue. Minimally processed to preserve what's valuable. Then cryogenically frozen in their own FDA-registered lab.

The science of regenerative medicine is being studied thoroughly as a method to restore function and balance in the body's systems. It is the science of living cells being used to potentially regenerate or facilitate the repair of cells damaged by disease, genetics, injury, or simple aging by stimulating the body's own repair mechanisms.

Cord Blood Collection

The collection, preservation, and storage of cord blood is a process that requires precision throughout each step. Everything from how the stem cells are obtained to how they are stored is precisely monitored.

> **Step 1:** Umbilical cord is clamped and cut from the baby after birth. This is already a part of the majority of births in North America and worldwide. Currently, in many locations, women sign a waver agreeing to have the umbilical cord either thrown away or donated.

> **Step 2:** Use a collection kit to obtain and pack the umbilical cord blood. This must be done as soon as possible. If the umbilical cord blood is donated, physicians are required to use the collection immediately after birth.

> **Step 3:** Within twenty-four hours, blood must be sent to the lab for testing and cryopreservation. Specific requirements for storage and transportation are set out in the guidelines for each cord blood bank.

> **Step 4:** Testing is completed to ascertain consistency in quality of the cord blood. More than fifty tests are done to ensure safe products for patients. Oftentimes, mothers are screened during pregnancy.

Step 5: The stem cells are processed using a new, patented technology to produce the maximum number of stem cells per sample.

Step 6: The stem cells are stored in liquid nitrogen.

Terrence's Story—Crippled with Arthritis

"For more than twenty-five years, I was practically crippled by arthritis. For some of that time, it was manageable. Though I was on medication for twelve years, it stopped working. Over about two months, the medication that was keeping me comfortable gradually worked less and less every day.

"And then everything was reduced to what other people could do for me. I was in daily pain; I couldn't walk at all, and I needed help for everything. Unfortunately, I was not the right size to need help from anyone.

"I was quite overweight, and I was often out of breath. My blood pressure was climbing, and my overall health was really bad. It took at least two people to help me up or get me mobile.

"Around this time, I lost contact with my family for a time. My daughter was mad at me for not taking care of myself, or her. Because of all of this, I didn't get to see my grandchildren for a period of time, and it was really hard.

"My family had had enough, and no one wanted to watch me suffer, so instead, they just ignored me unless I harassed them. So many of these issues built up over time, but they were all surrounding the same issue.

"Once I found out about stem cell therapy, it seemed like an answer coming in from the fog. It was never hard to talk me into it, as (1) I do not trust doctors who do not take time to talk to me, and (2) this was the first time I was given videos and other information that directly related to my health. It was scientific evidence showing how this new therapy could help my specific condition.

"I was blown away. When I got there, my defenses were up, as I am always ready to be talked into some treatment or medication. I was ready to berate them with questions, so I was in for a surprise when they answered all my questions before I got a chance to ask.

"They told me it would take about three months after having stem cell therapy to see any improvement, and they didn't promise anything. I forget the number, but there is a percentage of people who see no results at all.

"That was not the case for me, though, as I started noticing improvement immediately. My pain slowly got better, and day after day, I was able to do so much more than before."

Safety and Simplicity

More than 300,000 people have had stem cell therapy, with no adverse effects. It is a simple and convenient regenerative therapy that is evolving to benefit more and more conditions every year.

By using your own natural healing properties to lead to a better quality of life, this process combines engineering, clinical translation, and cellular therapy. The choice to use umbilical cord-sourced stem cells has a lot to do with safety and simplicity.

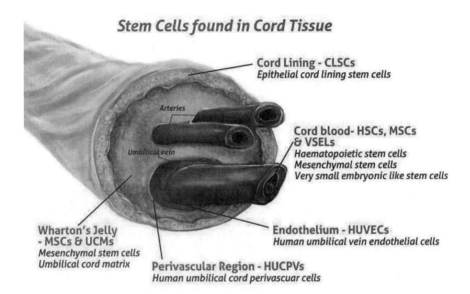

Stem Cells found in Cord Tissue

Cord Lining - CLSCs
Epithelial cord lining stem cells

Arteries

Cord blood- HSCs, MSCs & VSELs
Haematopoietic stem cells
Mesenchymal stem cells
Very small embryonic like stem cells

Umbilical vein

Wharton's Jelly - MSCs & UCMs
Mesenchymal stem cells
Umbilical cord matrix

Endothelium - HUVECs
Human umbilical vein endothelial cells

Perivascular Region - HUCPVs
Human umbilical cord perivascuar cells

The umbilical cord is the transportation center by which nutrients are passed between mother and baby. It is a long tube, full of blood vessels that connect the baby's stomach to the placenta inside the uterus.

The umbilical cord contains the following:

- A vein that passes oxygen and nutrients from mother to child through the bloodstream
- Two arteries that bring back waste and carbon dioxide to the bloodstream of the mother

There is a sticky substance surrounding all the blood cells called *Wharton's jelly*. This substance contains a high quantity of stem cells. Surrounding the Wharton's jelly is the *amnion*, a protective membrane that keeps everything contained.

The blood that is contained within the umbilical cord is highly oxygenated and rich in nutrients. As the umbilical cord is the lifeline to the baby, it contains a high concentration of young, regenerative cells.

As blood is transferred from the placenta to the fetus for nine months, it passes on many growth factors necessary for the birth of a healthy baby, including the following:

- Stem cells
- Immune cells
- Progenitor cells
- Proteins and growth factors

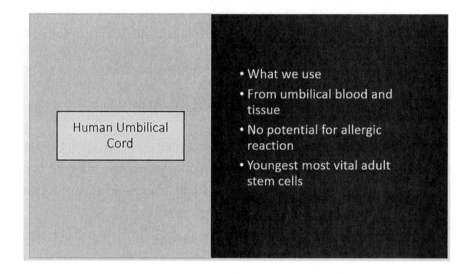

Although stem cells may be isolated from several locations such as umbilical cord blood and tissue, as well as adult tissues, the umbilical cord cells provide the most benefit and the least damage.

In 2005, a report was published by the National Academy of Sciences encouraging all medical centers to provide information to new parents about the benefits of cord blood banking. Legislation is now being investigated to ensure physicians and mothers have adequate information for donating and banking umbilical cord blood stem cells, after the child has been born.

Stem cells are considered *naïve cells,* which have the capacity to divide indefinitely. As such, they are able to change any cell in the body and adapt as necessary. This ability to differentiate was what first got stem cells noticed.

As scientists discovered their versatility, more and more uses for stem cell therapy were developed. Each type of stem cell works in its own way to help with regeneration and healing.

The mesenchymal stem cells (MSCs) are particularly beneficial and defined by an ability to do the following:

- Express surface molecules
- Differentiate between similar cells
- Heal and repair injured tissue
- Manage immune response
- Secrete proteins

These stem cells are the most versatile and most commonly found within the umbilical cord. It is a win-win situation as the mesenchymal stem cells are more likely adapt to the exact needs of the patient.

Regenerative medicine includes a vast array of products designed to naturally heal and repair the body. The more research that is done into the tiny, interrelated aspects of the healing power of the body, the more common regenerative health care is becoming. Stem cells play an integral role in healing and repair.

Umbilical cord blood contains stem cells, growth factors, and immune cells that are immature as they must be compatible to baby and mother. This makes them ideal for donor cells as the recipient patient is more likely to have successful results with cells that are so versatile.

For our stem cell therapy, we use several labs for regenerative medicine product (that comes from human umbilical cord tissue) that uses a patented technology to produce greater viability in cells.

As well, the product is isolated in a sterile environment and tested for blood-borne pathogens to assure safety. The product contains millions of cells in a vial, as demonstrated by AO/PI staining. It is positive for cell surface markers that suggest there are MSCs present in the total cell population and HSCs (hematopoietic stem cells).

The product is a regenerative medicine product that has many viable cells that may aid in host repair and healing. The scientific literature abounds with data illustrating that these products may be beneficial for many trauma and pain conditions.

Sally's Story—Torn Meniscus

"About five years ago, I had surgery, and it was supposed to be relatively routine. I had a torn meniscus. It was really starting to get to me, and I thought after recovering from surgery everything would get back to normal.

"It seemed like a routine thing people had done at my age. I had three or four close friends who had surgery and went back to work and lived active lives. At the time, I saw no reason why it would be different for me.

"But it was. After surgery, I got worse. The pain intensified immediately after surgery and never seemed to level off. I was unbalanced and always falling, which led me to not want to go anywhere. Besides, I could hardly walk anyway.

"We have a three-story house, and I had to walk up two flights of stairs to go to bed every day. There came a time when I just couldn't do it any longer.

"When my own house became a struggle to live in, I started to lose hope a little bit. No one seemed to understand why I wasn't improving. All my active friends seemed to think I just needed to walk more but what they didn't understand is I physically couldn't do it.

"It was excruciating agony pretty much all the time. And every doctor I went to only wanted me to go through more surgery. By that point, I didn't trust anything they told me, and I told a few of them that I thought they only wanted me to have surgery to line their pocketbooks or pay for their next holiday.

"To top it off, I found out I was allergic to titanium, so any surgery with implants was totally not going to happen. From that point on, I always said that I was allergic to doctors as well. They caused an adverse reaction that I could no longer shake.

"At the time, the only thing that would help was water therapy, because it took the pressure off. When I was submerged, it was the only time I got any relief from my pain.

"Before my chronic pain disabled me, I was a first responder in the health-care field. I knew what to look for with regard to my health-care options, but I was beyond fed up with what I was being offered.

"Then one day, kind of out of nowhere, I came across some information about stem cell therapy. So I spent a lot of time looking for information and researching all aspects of the science and research behind it. Everything made sense, and I had no concerns about the possibilities.

"When I made an appointment and finally had a meeting with the medical team, I was blown away by the professionalism of the entire office. They were not afraid of answering any of my questions, and I never got the impression that they were trying to sell me something.

"I was onboard and ready to try the stem cell therapy, and I was so relieved to have found out about the option. Immediately afterward, I felt improvement in movement. I am free again, truly free.

"Beforehand, I couldn't walk. We go to Disneyland every year with the great-grandchildren, and the last two years, I had to use a power chair. It was the first year I had to sit back and watch, instead of participating.

"At the same time, sitting in the chair all day was hot. I got so stiff and uncomfortable, and it was the first year that I really did not enjoy the holiday. It was awful. And remembering it through the few pictures I have is like seeing a whole other person.

"That trip is coming up again, and I am eager to stretch my legs and follow the magic in the kid's eyes, instead of being crippled with pain.

"Anyone who asks me knows I would do it again in a heartbeat, and I have already recommended stem cell therapy to at least six other people."

Food and Drug Administration

The FDA provides criteria regarding human cells, tissues, and cellular- and tissue-based products, manufacturers, health-care providers, and FDA staff. The current Title 21 of the Code of Federal Regulation is the portion of the Code of Federal Regulations that governs food and drugs within the United States for the Food and Drug Administration (FDA), the Drug Enforcement Administration (DEA), and the Office of National Drug Control Policy (ONDCP).

The criteria are listed within the regulations to ensure minimal manipulation and homologous use of biological substances. The definitions of key terms that are related to the industry and concerned industry stakeholders are also included.

It is the intent of the FDA to provide guidance to improve an understanding of the appropriate use of stem cells. These regulatory criteria apply to the following:

- Manufacturers
- Health-care providers
- Educators
- And other professionals involved in stem cell therapy.

The FDA also maintains enforcement discretion under limited conditions with respect to investigating the use of stem cell therapy for approved therapies. The comprehensive guidelines are detailed as to all aspects of the process, including the use of the following:

- Stem cells
- Tissue-based products (HCT/Ps)
- Adipose tissue
- Any substance consisting of human cells

All tissues that are intended for implantation, transplantation, infusion, or transfer into a human must be closely monitored for safety and health concerns.

The FDA uses a tiered, risk-based approach to the regulation of stem cells. As well, the FDA is authorized to enforce federal laws and regulations contained in the following:

1. Federal Food, Drug, and Cosmetic Act (FD&C Act)
2. Public Health Service Act (PHS Act)

Any therapies that use stem cells or meet the specific criteria must follow the regulations applied to that category. In developing the therapies, the focus must always be on public health.

Concerns about adequate regulation are eased as the FDA has regulations that can prevent these outcomes:

- Communicable disease
- Contamination
- Unsafe or ineffective product
- Unknown origin of stem cells
- Misleading information
- False claims

In this way, the function, safety, and effectiveness of the products are protected. Patients are assured of a level of professionalism and that everyone experiences the same process and procedure. The intention is to protect the people who seek these therapies for health improvement.

Disclaimer

The U.S. Food and Drug Administration (FDA) has stated that stem cells, like other medical products that are intended to treat, cure, or prevent diseases, generally require FDA approval before they can be marketed.

FDA has not approved any stem cell-based products for use, other than cord blood-derived hematopoietic progenitor cells (blood-forming stem cells) for certain indications. If you are considering stem cell treatment, you should be aware that stem cell therapies have enormous promise, but the science in each use is still in the developmental stage.

Professional judgment and expertise is needed in using stem cells for any therapeutic use, and we urge anyone embarking on the use of stem cell therapies to consult the national health databases to evaluate current information from clinical trials, and the FDA websites on human tissue should also be consulted to get its current evaluation of any therapy.

By following the rules and requirements of the FDA and focusing on the healthful results shown by recent scientific studies, health-care professionals can offer some hope to their patients for a better life to come.

The Future of Stem Cell Therapy

Imagine a world where healing centers focused on the entire system of the body in an attempt to preserve and improve quality of life. In this world, patients would be viewed as partners in health, and their feedback and involvement as crucial to their well-being.

This future world is being set into motion, based on the hard work and determination of scientists, doctors, and patients alike. Governments and regulatory boards are ensuring research can continue by placing laws and procedures to protect the scientific process.

In this world of holistic healing, regenerative medicine is at the forefront of options for patients. Prior to receiving prescriptions for lifelong medications or undergoing irreversible surgeries and other treatment, patients are being offered stem cell therapy, if it is applicable to them.

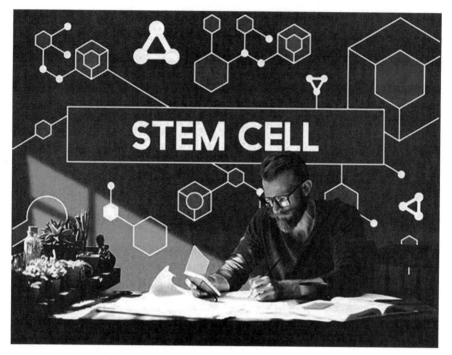

Future doctors will have the decades of scientific research and clinical applications to use as a guide for their practices. Medical colleges will move away from a do-no-harm mentality to one of constant attention to the healing properties of the body. Stem cell therapy will be studied and practiced and reiterated to med students as a go-to procedure for a vast array of conditions.

Having studied and practiced stem cell therapy during their years of education, doctors will be confident in offering it as a primary solution to their patient's ailments. From this position of prevention, people will suffer less as they will not be subjected to needless and painful treatment.

Imagine a world where stem cell therapy changed the way we view health care. Not only are people healthier because the focus is on healing the body, but they are also more conscious of how the various aspects of their health work together.

In this world, accepting of regenerative medicine, some unrelated wellness issues are addressed with the increased use of stem cell therapy:

- Addiction to prescription painkillers subsides as people find a more permanent solution.
- Life expectancy and quality of life increase as health issues are detected and prevented.
- Health-care costs are reduced as fewer major surgeries are required.
- Hospitals become health centers focused on holistic healing.
- Wait times for emergency medical care are reduced as fewer patients require care.
- People begin to take a proactive approach to their health as they understand how the body's processes work.
- Science and research continue to make advances, nearly eradicating the top causes of death worldwide as the regenerative properties of stem cells are more clearly understood.
- Other sources of regenerative medicine are discovered as people become more open to new ways of healing the body.
- Instead of treating the sick, medical professionals are trained to have an outlook of maintaining and rejuvenating health in their patients.

Although this is all speculation in an imaginary world, a lot of it is not far off. People are realizing the power of stem cell therapy, and it aligns with their views of a more-natural healing path. Advances in regenerative medicine will continue, and in the years to come, people may look back and see that many of these outcomes have come to pass.

Stem cell therapy—using umbilical cord blood as a source— is seeing more and more use as scientific studies show promising results. Following the strategic tactics used to ensure safe and ethical procedures will help research progress in a slow and steady manner.

Sourcing umbilical cord blood in a way that ensures proper testing and screening allows for the youngest, most effective cells to be made available from something that is, for the most part, going to waste.

The hesitation regarding stem cell therapy is lessening as people come to understand the science behind the source and the subject. As a natural healing technique, it is offering hope, as can be seen from previously skeptical patients and the studies, whose numbers speak for themselves.

CHAPTER 4

What Stem Cell Therapy Can Offer

Hope, Healing, Happiness

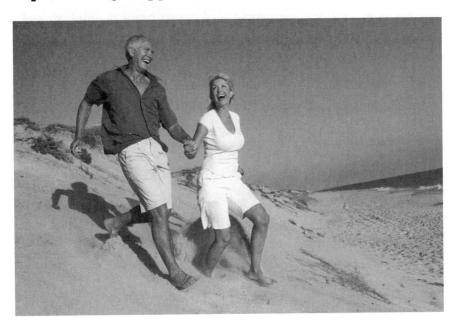

Stem cell therapy has moved beyond the controversial, and into the realm of proven science. The results of stem cell therapy are showing benefits in such a wide range of health issues, and each patient's story speaks for itself. As new research is being studied in a broad scope of areas, vast improvements in this healing therapy are expected.

After looking into the science of stem cell therapy, we are now going to go into how this heals the body. From there, we will get specific about some of the main conditions that have been studied and researched with scrutiny.

Stem cell therapy is bringing hope, healing, and happiness to patients who previously suffered from conditions that could only be monitored. Throughout this chapter, we are going to share how this holistic health process is providing a new way for people with chronic conditions.

This is not a book for people looking to prove a point; this is a book for people who want to see what proven results look like through the research and lives of people who have experienced it. The science behind the therapy has been happening and researched for more than a decade.

Stem cell therapy advancements are being studied worldwide. Doctors, educators, and researchers are working together to inform and educate people on the hundreds of disorders and diseases that are being improved through stem cell therapy.

So many of the varied benefits that result from stem cell therapy can be summed up in the following categories:

1. Hope

"When my granddaughter was born, I couldn't hold her. My elbow hurt so bad I couldn't lift a glass to my lips. It broke my heart. The morning after my stem cell therapy, I remember lifting a glass of orange juice to my lips, and I had hope."

– CAROL

So many people lose hope when traditional medical procedures and surgeries don't relieve their symptoms. The calm, healing nature of this therapy gives people hope for a different quality of life.

The noninvasive nature of the procedure provides a stress-free environment. Many patients see results quite quickly afterward. For many, when they finally see some improvement in their condition, it gives them the hope they need to keep going in the direction of a healthy life.

A big part of healing and overall health is a mental or emotional well-being. Hope ignites these feelings and encourages ongoing wellness.

2. Happiness

"It didn't hurt to laugh anymore. I couldn't believe what a difference it made to feel joy without pain. It was like a cloud lifted."

– Daryl

Our mental and emotional health is affected by our physical health. When physical conditions and symptoms are present long term, they can cause mental health issues such as these:

- Depression
- Suicide
- Anger and irritability
- Lack of clarity
- Inability to focus
- Mental fog
- Sadness
- Violent outbursts

When the physical condition is improved, or cellular structures regenerated, the healing is also emotional and mental. Reducing pain and physical restriction allows people the comfort to live in happiness. Although happiness is subjective to each individual's circumstances, it is closely tied to health. Seen as an important goal to achieve, through healing, happiness can vastly improve overall life quality.

3. Healing

"The stem cell therapy was the beginning of a total transformation for me. It felt like a system restart, allowing me to become new and improved. On a spiritual level, I could almost feel it working with my body toward a more healing being in my entire wellness."

- SANDRA

The more we learn about the human body and how health happens, the better we can balance the systems involved. Stem cell therapy takes the science of the systems and provides regeneration, restoration, and relief.

The process of healing, regardless of what area of the body it is in, happens following these same basic steps:

Step 1: Alarm
- Depending on the condition, the body reacts to the negative stimulus in the form of nerve signals to the brain.

Step 2: Response
- The brain sends out an appropriate response via the immune system or other bodily functions.

Step 3: Reaction

- During this step, the body fights whatever is harming it. This is an ongoing process as the location and type of health issue determines to what capacity it can attack.

Step 4: Intervention

- Often the condition will continue to cause degeneration or other symptoms as the body fights a stalemate battle. From there, the patient might seek out assistance from the medical community as the body becomes weakened and unstable.

Step 5: Healing

- Eventually, the patient, with the help of the health-care providers, must find a pathway to improvement, either through medication, surgery, or another treatment or procedure.

Stem cells are designed for healing. It is their cellular purpose, and when they are taken from umbilical cord blood that would otherwise be discarded, the healing process is beneficial from all perspectives.

When your body heals, the pain and other symptoms go away. By working with your body, you activate the process to improve your overall health, rather than use surgery or medication to mask the problem.

Rob's Story—Spinal Cord Injury

"Okay, I am not a testimonial guy. I am not a natural health guy either. In fact, everyone who knows me thought I was joking when I said stem cell therapy is what made the difference. Sure, they saw the improvement, but they didn't believe me right away.

"I'll tell you right now, the first thing I asked was how much is this going to cost me? It's not covered by insurance, of course, so I figured it must be a money-grab. That was one thing that surprised me—I could actually afford it.

"When I had my bike accident, I thought I would bounce back like I had when I was younger. But it didn't happen that way. What used to be on-and-off back pain turned into a spinal cord injury that changed everything.

"Suddenly I was an old guy. I couldn't ride; I was even starting to use a walker. So then, I didn't want to go anywhere because I didn't want to be the guy with the walker everyone felt sorry for. I groaned whenever I moved, and I was getting angrier and angrier.

"I was really skeptical and figured all of the testimonials were made up, but I gave it a try anyway. For the most part, it was old habits die hard, and I wanted to make sure I had tried everything before surgery.

"When I started noticing an improvement, I tried to convince myself it was all in my head. But within five or six weeks, I couldn't deny the improvement. I hadn't needed to use the walker in close to a month. I was sleeping again, which made a huge improvement on my mood.

"Everyone who knew me was shocked at the improvement and started asking me what I did. As time went on, it was like the chronic pain caused by my spinal cord injury had been nothing more than a bad dream.

"Now I am back and better than ever, and the only anger I feel is at how long it took me to find out about stem cell therapy."

—ROB W.

The Body's Ability to Heal

Stem cell therapy is the result of the body's natural ability to heal itself. Although many patients have inspiring stem cell stories, they are actually science-based and quite common. Our physiological systems have regeneration built into them.

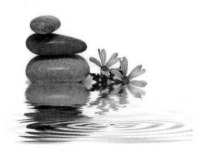

Our cells are dying, and new ones are growing at all times, so healing is not a new subject. It is the basic function of our bodies to replace nonfunctioning cells with functioning ones, to manage issues, and overcome viruses. As old cells degenerate, new ones take their place. We see it most obviously in our fingernails and hair.

The top ways the body naturally heals itself are as follows:

- The liver can regenerate every 300 to 500 days and compensate for the loss of the gall bladder.
- Our skeletal system replaces itself entirely with new cells approximately every ten years.

- The surface layer of the skin (the epidermis) regenerates every two weeks as it is often damaged.
- Some cells have a longer life span than others, but all are replaced more than once during a person's life.
- Muscle cells from the ribs will be replaced after a little more than a decade.
- Red blood cells travel through the body for around 120 days before they are recycled in the spleen and replaced.
- The epithelial cells that line the stomach must regenerate much more quickly due to the harsh nature of their responsibility. These cells last only around five days.
- Hair grows approximately a half-inch every three months, but what is interesting is that process slows if the patient is unwell in other areas of their body.
- It takes six months to completely regrow a fingernail, and toenails take longer, often up to eighteen months because more stress and pressure is put on that area of the body.

These are just a few examples of regeneration that naturally occurs in the body. Every day, new cells are being grown by the body for many different systems and reasons. As science catches up with the human body's natural tendencies, we will learn more and more about the interplay between the systems.

Just as the body naturally heals from cuts, bruises, and common maladies, so too, can it regenerate in other ways. Stem cell therapy works to enhance this process by putting the healing cells right where they are needed.

Every single university is doing research on stem cells, perfecting and ensuring the efficacy of stem cell therapy. For different patients, undergoing different therapies, for different conditions across the board, stem cell therapy is being studied carefully.

A new study from The Ohio State University Wexner Medical Center is providing more insight into how the body heals itself and how stem cells can increase this regeneration. The research shows that immune cells of the adult body may behave like stem cells and generate new cell types required for wound healing.

According to that study: *"These findings show, for the first time, that immune cells are a major source of collagen-producing fibroblasts at the site of wound healing. The study also provides a new avenue to manage inflammation by converting inflammatory cells to other cell types."*

As scientific research continues to shed light on how the body regenerates, the parallels as to how stem cell therapy can boost this process will become clearer. Each study adds to the evidence of the efficacy of the procedure.

At the same time, each of the sources and types of stem cell therapy offer different levels of efficacy. In some ways, it is like comparing apples and oranges, and patients might become frustrated their results are impeded by their choice in therapy.

For simplicity's sake, let's compare different types of stem cell therapies to televisions. Stay with me for a minute, and it will make sense. Think back with me to the first TV you ever watched. If you are like me, it was a large, square box with a small, fuzzy screen, and it was probably black and white. The way I remember it, there were only one or two channels, and you would sometimes have to knock on its side to get the picture to stop jumping. There was also an antenna that you would have to move back and forth to try to get good reception. If you could make out everyone's face, it was a good day.

What I am getting at here is that those old-fashioned, black-and-white TV sets are what bone marrow and adipose stem cells are like in regenerative medicine. They are age-dependant, and although they may work well enough to see the picture, it might not be enough to provide a solution to the health condition.

On the other hand, umbilical cord stem cells replicate every twenty-four hours, which we have already discussed. So umbilical cord stem cell therapy is like a 3-D, 72-inch, flat-screen smart-TV experience, with every additional option available, compared to a 15-inch, black-and-white pixelated screen.

When it comes down to it, there is no comparison because one provides a quality and consistency far superior to the other. If you want to maximize healing and regeneration, you must use the highest-quality therapy you can find.

Knee Pain

The what, when, and why of knee pain is so common it is a topic for another book, or series of books. However, since so many patients who seek out stem cell therapy struggle with knee pain, we would do well to touch on a few things.

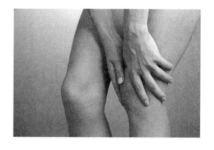

One of the reasons knee pain is so frequent in people from all walks of life is because it is one of the most used joints. Almost every movement we make or every position we are in requires the joint effort of multiple tendons, muscles, and bones in the knee.

A person does not even have to be extremely athletic to have knee pain, though it is one of the most common athletic injuries. Simply sitting, standing, bending, reaching, and crouching on a day-to-day basis can be severely restricted by knee pain.

These are some of the many different causes of pain in the knee, and which often become chronic:

- Fracture
- Torn meniscus
- Inflammation
- Tendonitis
- Mechanical problems
- Accident or injury
- Arthritis
- Genetic abnormalities
- Excess weight or obesity

Knee problems are also some of the most complicated and expensive medical conditions because of the complexity of the situation. Knee replacements can cost upwards of $45,000 to $65,000 for the surgery alone.

Millions of people suffer from knee pain caused by arthritis as well. Add up the other causes and this number increases substantially. As surgery, injections, and medication fail to improve knee pain for patients, more and more people are seeking answers elsewhere.

Now we are seeing, more and more, that the cost and trauma of surgery, as well as recovery time can be avoided with stem cells. Stem cells modulate inflammation. Stem cells help so much, because they regulate the process of the immune system attacking itself. Reducing inflammation around the joints, especially in the knee. At the same time, the regenerating properties encourage new growth of cushioning, connective tissue.

This is just one example of many that shows why stem cell therapy is being called the healing revolution, and it is only just getting started. Now that the science has proven itself, there is no telling what new advancements will be discovered.

Cheryl's Story—Weakness and Knee Pain

"I always had bad knees. When I was just a kid, my family would tease me that I sounded like an old person as they were always cracking when I got up or sat down. Now I am not sure if it is genetic; I was just born with it, or it was some sort of curse to be different.

"What I did know is I didn't want to be anyone's charity. For so long, I either ignored the pain or just didn't do anything. What was the point when it hurt all the time anyway.

"Unfortunately for me, it was a vicious cycle. Because my knees caused me trouble, I was never very active. So the older I got, the more weight I started to gain. The extra weight I continued to put on turned around and caused more difficulty on my knees.

"For a few years, I got around mostly by motorized scooter. Even walking to the door or bending to tie my shoes would leave me out of breath. And there came a point where I no longer enjoyed my outings because the struggle to get ready and out the door was exhausting.

"People think when you hurt all the time you will eventually get used to it. I thought that, for sure. I remember when my knees would get bad, I would think that eventually the pain would be so commonplace that I wouldn't notice it any more. Well, that was a pipe dream. The pain definitely does not go away. If anything, it gets worse.

"When you get no relief, it wears your body to the point of exhaustion. You are tired, but cannot sleep. You ache and cannot get comfortable. All because of pain.

"Another thing about getting older is how much harder everything is on your body. My doctors had been trying to talk me into another surgery, and I was really hesitant. I doubted it would do any good.

"When I came down with the common cold, I couldn't shake it. It took me out, and I was sicker than I had ever felt before. It was like my immune system was done. It was a bit of a wake-up call as I was bed ridden and too weak to function for weeks on end.

"While in bed recovering, I finally knew I would recover; I decided 'I am no longer living in pain without working to improve it.' There was no way I was going to have surgery; I felt too old to bounce back. No, I had to find something easier on me.

"Stem cell therapy came across my path while I was looking for anything that might help me. Of course, a friend of a friend had tried it, and it worked great. But I needed more information than what this acquaintance was providing.

"So I signed up for a seminar that was supposed to educate me about stem cells. It didn't cost anything, and I came out of the seminar, after it was done, in a state of shock. Stem cell therapy wasn't anything like what I expected.

"The seminar provided straightforward, exact info and research to back up all the claims. It was one of those rare moments where they answer all your objections before you make them. Hands down, it was the most detailed, non-condescending, and reassuring experience.

"Afterward, there was no pressure or sales tactics like you sometimes find at these sorts of things. It was very welcoming

and reassuring, and I would have taken part in the therapy right there if I could.

"But anyway, I made an appointment, and there happened to be a cancellation, so I got in right away. It was such an amazing experience, and every doctor and staff member I encountered brought positivity and rejuvenation to my life.

"After I had the therapy, I didn't notice a difference right away. My knees continued to bother me, but I was starting to notice increased stamina and less weakness. I figured it must be my imagination because it was not like a night-and-day switch.

"During the initial consult, I had been encouraged to make a list of my symptoms that bothered me the most. Afterward, I was to cross off the ones that went away or became more manageable. Over time, I eventually crossed the following symptoms off of my list:

- *Weakness in my legs*
- *Insomnia*
- *Inability to walk*
- *Constant pain*
- *Depression*

"It was a gradual improvement that I could only describe as slow repair. After a few weeks, I couldn't doubt it any longer.

"Then one day, I was out running errands. It was a totally non-special day. I think I was waiting in line at the bank or something. And a light went off, and I realized as I had been going from place to place, I was thinking about what I needed to do next, what was for supper, and plans for later in the week.

> *"For once, I was not standing there in pain, wondering how to get the bare minimum done. It was like a freedom from a cage I didn't realize I was in."*
>
> —CHERYL N.

Transforming Lives Using Cells for Medicine

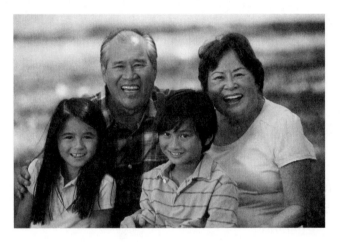

Cells have been used for medicine since the first transplant over a hundred years ago. Since then, stem cell therapy is a game changer for the health-care system. Instead of managing symptoms, it gets to the heart of the problem and offers a solution.

Healing the body is a process that sometimes requires outside influences. In the same way, as humans, we work together or serve to segregate. Using stem cell therapy to boost regeneration is like giving your body the gift of healing.

> *"New research suggests that perhaps we should consider stem cells one of the secrets to a longer life."*
>
> —TIME MAGAZINE

At the time of our birth, it is estimated that we have over 20,000 stem cells. Close to 1,300 of them are active at one time. As the body ages, the cells degenerate, leaving less stem cells available for regeneration.

This points to the fact that there may be a limit on the number of times a cell can divide. Once it has reached that limit, it is no longer active. Since it has been discovered that, the older people are, the fewer stem cells people have, it has been postulated that stem cells might be a requirement of life.

In a way, stem cell therapy acts as the body's repair kit, speeding up the length of time it takes for injuries or wounds to heal. Using cells to enhance the biological functions is a way that naturally occurs as a whole-healing approach.

As people take control over their options, they begin to see that this is not new. Mounting research continues to show optimistic results when using stem cell therapy for the following:

- Inflammation
- Immune system issues
- Degeneration
- Functional abnormalities
- Neurological damage
- Bone and tissue damage
- Cardiovascular disease
- Joint pain

Stem cells divide quickly and communicate effectively—it is their purpose and how human life grows from the beginning. Using the scientific research and studies compiled on the subject, it becomes clear why we use umbilical cord stem cell therapy.

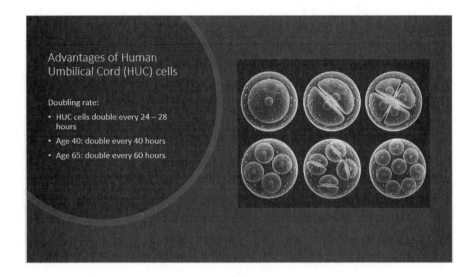

Every patient we encounter appreciates the professional process, where they move through our medical facility with guidance through every step of the way. It is in this way we prepare them for the potential possibilities of stem cell therapies.

Many times, people want to rush to the end result, having their life transformed. Yet still, we take it step by step to make sure everyone has adequate information:

Step 1: Education
This is when we define what stem cells are in terms that makes sense. We also go over the properties and purpose of stem cells, specifically in regard to the condition and   symptoms of the individual patient.

Step 2: Science
Next, we take it a bit deeper, helping people understand what is meant by regenerative medicine and stem cell therapy, and show them some of the research and studies that have been

done. Once again, we focus on similar instances to what the patient is experiencing and provide a background knowledge of the condition itself. This provides a clear picture to the patient as to what their body is experiencing.

Step 3: Therapies

The types of stem cell therapies available are described with a focus on what we do in our medical practice and why. Sharing other patient's experiences and providing details of what improvements are common are essential aspects of this step.

Step 4: Review

Once the patient understands everything involved, we make it a point to review science, research, and safety of stem cell therapy. Here we answer questions and make sure all the information is clearly understood.

Step 5: Patient's Choice

At this stage, the patient has all of the information required to determine whether stem cell therapy is a good personal fit. We encourage patients to make the choice that feels right, and provide a summary of the options that best fit their situations.

Your Body's Regenerating Factor

Just as your hair and fingernails grow, your body has a natural ability to regenerate itself; the same is true for all body systems. Some of them are just harder to notice than others. Regeneration is part of regrowth and how we came into existence to begin with.

Using the same practices that naturally occur in the body, the science, research, and potential of regenerative medicine is changing the way healing is looked at. By offering a beginner's understanding of stem cell therapy, patients can decide for themselves.

It can be difficult to illustrate the remarkable journey of stem cells, from the umbilical cord, where the donor stem cells are taken, to the specific area on the recipient's body, when received. And what comes before all of that is how the stem cells regenerate, by design.

Some of the regenerating properties of stem cells are seen in conditions which *improve* after therapy. This is especially true for chronic conditions with a high medication rate. The regenerating factors of stem cells are breaking new ground, with many different areas of the body gaining distinct benefits such as these:

- Reduced pain
- Increased functionality, range of motion, and flexibility
- Improved sleep quality
- Reduced risk for future injuries
- Decreased nerve damage
- Increased collagen
- New tissue growth
- Prevention of formation of scar tissue
- Reduced hair loss
- Return to normal activities

That last one, return to normal activities, is so huge for most people. They do not even realize what was missing, until they get it back. Half the reason I am writing this book is that it breaks my heart to know how many people are living lives in pain, not thinking they can have a better quality of life.

For many of these people, improving even one thing on their extensive lists of symptoms would be enough to give them a reason to continue their healing. The power of regenerative medicine is strong enough to bring health care to a holistic new level.

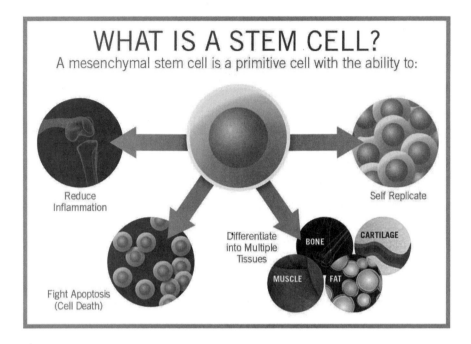

Really, it all goes back to the hope we talked about in the beginning of the chapter. And that hope is closely tied to healing and happiness. The knowledge we have of regenerative properties and how health therapies are adapting to share this benefit is *hope made real.*

Jason's Story—Autoimmune Disorder

"When I was diagnosed with an undetermined autoimmune disorder, to say I was feeling a lack of reassurance was an understatement. Every appointment I had, the doctors seemed to fumble around the numbers and my levels, which meant nothing to me. At the same time, my health conditions and the symptoms I was having seemed to mean nothing to them.

"It was like we were speaking different languages. I had never heard about autoimmune issues before. Sure, I had heard some names like these:

- *ALS (amyotrophic lateral sclerosis)*
- *Crohn's*
- *Parkinson's*
- *Hashimoto's*
- *Irritable Bowel Syndrome (IBS)*

"Still, I never grasped the connection, until I was told my health issues were actually an autoimmune issue. Because it was undetermined, and I did not have one of the above listed or any other named disease, there was no category to put me in. This made it hard to treat according to the doctors.

"For me, it just left me baffled, and I realized how much "modern medicine" still doesn't know. Since I couldn't even look up my condition or tell people what was wrong with me, I felt like a fraud. As though, if it was unnamed, I was making it up.

"The problem was it took me years to understand what any of it even meant. See, no doctor ever sat down with me and discussed what an autoimmune issue was caused by and how it usually progressed.

"Instead, they talked about managing numbers and different prescription dosages. Mostly, they told me what symptoms I could expect as my condition deteriorated.

"After a while, I went through a really dark time where I didn't care about myself at all. Before I retired, I had moved to a new city to take a higher-paying job. All of my family and friends were thousands of miles away.

"So I stopped contacting them, stopped going anywhere, and stayed in a painful blanket of symptoms. I watched too much TV, but didn't pay attention to any of it. Then I got a wake-up call.

"Two people close to me lost their lives, one right after another. Both were sudden and unexpected, and now I had to go home. I still had family and people I loved in the world, and it kind of shook me awake to realize I was letting my life drift by.

"Of course, some people in my life noticed a big difference in my health and overall well-being. One of them was my mom. Moms always know, and it is hard to lie to them. She was worried about me.

"I changed the subject though, because she had changed a lot, too—for the better. I hadn't seen her for a few years (and yes, I had plenty of excuses as to why not), but she looked wonderful. Last time we visited, I noticed she was starting to slow down, which in her late eighties is not surprising.

"Now though, she seemed younger or spryer or something. It was hard to pinpoint, but basically the opposite of what was happening to me. That is when she told me about stem cell therapy.

"She had learned about it when she had trouble with her hip. After choosing stem cell therapy, instead of a future hip replacement, she was thrilled with her overall improvement in health.

"If it was anyone other than my mom, I probably would have laughed it off or put it off to a placebo effect or something. But that woman was more skeptical than I was, and she was not one for dramatics. She was as straight-laced as they come, and right away, I knew I needed to look into it a little further.

"*The biggest reason I went through with stem cell therapy (of course, after everything checked out) was because, for the first time, I felt like I had some control over my own health. It wasn't going to be a huge ordeal that I had to recover from.*

"*From the moment I contacted the medical office, I felt like I was given choices, information, and hope. For once, I wasn't given the runaround.*

"*What I didn't expect is how quickly I would start to feel better after receiving stem cell therapy. It was almost immediate and lasted for months, until I felt like my old self again. I remember laughing with my mom in her kitchen while she waved her spoon at me and said she told me so.*

"*Looking back, it is crazy to me how simple it was. How the answer to my healing was in the form of a therapy that was efficient, effective, and affordable. And especially how desperate things had to get before I found it.*

"*Luckily, that seems to be changing, as since I have been getting better, I hear about stem cell therapy more and more. And that gives me hope too, that others will hear about this as an option so that they do not have to suffer any longer than necessary.*"

—JASON V.

A Family Affair

Earlier, I mentioned that so many doctors who provide stem cell therapy are patients of it themselves, as am I. Basically, once people understand how it works and see the results, well, it is straight-forward from there.

When health care professionals see the science and studies, they usually want to be involved in offering the therapy to others. They also often have multiple members of their family who listen to their advice.

It kind of goes hand in hand. Just like when you eat at a really great restaurant, and you want to tell everyone else about it. Or if you find a cool app that saves you time and money. People like to be on the cutting edge of what is new, and at the same time, share what is working with others.

In the same way, many people in the same family undergo stem cell therapy for different conditions. After seeing firsthand someone you love going from miserable and stuck in discomfort, and then after a simple procedure, to regaining a significant part of life is inspiring.

Jason's story is one of a patient finding out about stem cells through a family member, and I have heard a lot of people with similar stories. In fact, some of those similar stories come from my own family, as more than one of my family members have their own experiences and stories to tell.

If you go back to chapter 1, we talked about Mel Gibson's father. In that same interview, he talks about using stem cell therapy for his own health after seeing the remarkable difference it made for his father. Since then, he has come out publicly to recommend stem cell therapy.

So many others have done the same thing. It is so easy to see firsthand the simple effectiveness that stem cell therapy provides. The remarkable part is how many different applications and uses there are for the same therapy.

By simply altering the location of the procedure, we can target exactly the area the patient needs help with. Since our stem cells are young and viable, they get to work right away. Now patients who are thrilled with their results are reaching out to let others know how this treatment was finally the end to their pain and suffering.

When stem cell therapy was new, the efficacy was shared, for the most part, by word of mouth. As the years went on, with research and scientific findings continuing to show success of stem cell therapy, more and more people have realized how revolutionary it really is.

A Focus on Each Patient

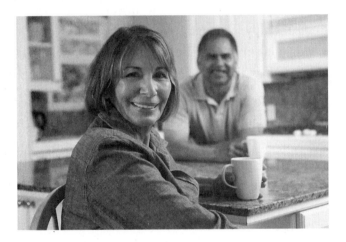

Stem cell therapy benefits overall health so much because stem cells modulate the healing process, helping regulate the body systems. Each individual patient might have various levels of severity of certain issues. In each case, the stem cell therapy helps in these ways:

- Lowers inflammation
- Reduces immune issues
- Helps the body adapt
- Provides regeneration and promotes regrowth
- Encourages natural healing processes

It is no secret that the most vocal supporters of stem cell therapy are those whose lives have changed significantly since seeing improvements in their condition after therapy. This includes many doctors who are now stem cell recipients themselves, as leaders embracing this relatively new in-clinic practice.

Many patients are getting older, so their stem cells are not as abundant or effective as they used to be. Stem cell therapy is helping these people rejuvenate and heal in remarkable ways.

What makes it unique is the patient's condition, and how stem cell therapy can target the exact spot where the problem is occurring. For many years, one of the mainstream medical treatments offered was to get cortisone injections. But cortisone injections are vastly different from stem cell therapy, because stem cells migrate to the exact areas of damage and inflammation. The difference to note is that cortisone causes degeneration, while stem cells support healing and regeneration.

It is our passion to help people heal. In following the research to the therapies that provide the most benefit, with the least side effects, we can give people access to the cutting edge of healing. When we talk to our patients and hear their stories, we get a chance to share with them what stem cell therapy can offer.

Full Disclaimer

The use of stem cells or stem cell-rich tissues, as well as the mobilization of stem cells by any means, e.g., pharmaceutical, mechanical, or herbal-nutrient based is not FDA approved to combat aging or to prevent, treat, cure, or mitigate any disease or medical condition mentioned in this book.

RegenHealthMed.com is a medical team—we are a collaboration of doctors of medicine (MDs), including orthopedic surgeons, and we are educators, teaching people about the benefits of stem cells.

This book and the information featured, showcased, or otherwise appearing in it is not to be used as a substitute for medical advice, diagnosis, or treatment of any health condition or problem. Those who read this book should not rely on information provided in it for their own health problems. Any questions regarding your own health should be addressed by your physician or other duly licensed health-care provider.

This book makes no guarantees, warranties, or express or implied representations whatsoever with regard to the accuracy, completeness, timeliness, comparative or controversial nature, or usefulness of any information contained or referenced on this website. This book and its owners and operators do not assume any risk whatsoever for your use of this book or the information posted herein.

Health-related information and opinions change frequently, and therefore, information contained in this book may be outdated, incomplete, or incorrect. All statements made about products, drugs, and such in this book have not been evaluated by the U.S. Food and Drug Administration (FDA). In addition, any testimonials appearing in this book are based on the experiences of a few people, and you are not likely to have similar results. Use of this book does not create an expressed or implied professional relationship.

In accordance with the Federal Trade Commission (FTC) guidelines concerning the use of endorsements and testimonials in advertising, please be aware of the following. Federal regulations require us to advise you that all reviews, testimonials, and/or endorsements of any kind reflect the personal experiences of those individuals who have expressed their own personal opinions, and those opinions and experiences may not be representative of what every consumer may personally experience with the endorsement.

All reviews and testimonials are the sole opinions, findings, and/or experiences of the people sharing their stories. These people are not compensated in any way.

These statements have not been evaluated by the U.S. Food and Drug Administration (FDA). We are required to inform you that there is no intention—implied or otherwise—that represents or infers that these statements be used in the cure, diagnosis, mitigation, treatment, and/or prevention of any disease.

These testimonials do not imply that similar results would or could happen for you. These testimonials are not intended to diagnose for specific illnesses or conditions, or be a treatment to eliminate diseases or other medical conditions or complications.

We make no medical claims as to the benefits of anything to improve medical conditions. We have to make the disclaimer our own and put a statement about the stories we used and not call them testimonials.

CHAPTER 5
Proven Therapies and Case Histories

Proven Therapies

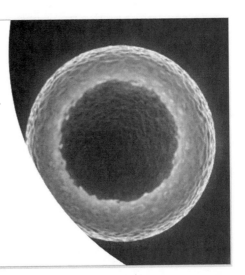

Stem Cell Therapy

- Direction healthcare is headed
- Used by athlete's for 10+ years
- Changes in rules & regulations have allowed stem cell therapy to be available at reasonable cost

When we talk about stem cell therapy, we must go from the very generic biological function of how stem cells work and why to very specific actions happening within each individual condition. Since the procedure and results are unique, depending on the *region* and the *reason*, we are going to break down the most common conditions that have seen proven results with stem cell therapy.

So in this chapter, I am going to go a little bit deeper into each of the conditions that are commonly seen in the patients with whom I talk who are seeking stem cell therapy. While each person experiences the condition differently, knowing the background and specifics of the condition itself provides a better understanding of all the options available to help you regain your health.

Some people find they have more than one condition on the list; others relate to one specific cause or symptom. Either way, I have broken down each condition into sections of related facts and information. You will see that each condition contains the following details:

1. **Definition:** A description about the condition in detail, including causes, symptoms, and treatment

2. **Causes and Symptoms:** How the condition makes you feel, and how it affects day-to-day life, as well as information on what the main causes of the condition are

3. **Anatomy:** An image of the affected area of the body to illustrate where the issues occur and provide a visual of how stem cell therapy can improve the condition

4. **Diagnosis and Treatment:** From how a condition is discovered and tested to what the medical system provides as a solution to control symptoms with medication or surgical repair or replacement

5. **When to Seek Help:** This one is important as it contains what to look for and when to seek immediate medical attention.

6. **Long-Term Outlook:** A description of how the condition will affect overall health from the outset and for years to come

7. **Why Stem Cell Therapy:** An explanation of how stem cell therapy works to improve symptoms and function, specifically in the area of concern for each condition

8. **Case Study:** A patient's personal experience with stem cell therapy shared in their words

9. **Science:** Research, studies, and journal articles about stem cell therapy for each specific condition

This section is meant to be a reference to you, so you can better understand your condition and symptoms and how stem cell therapy might work in your situation.

Knowledge is the first step toward healing, so understanding how and why a condition occurs and what exactly it is doing to the body gives insight into possible solutions for healing.

Although it is a relatively new therapy, stem cell therapy was discovered as a result of earlier research and study into cellular structure and function. Having knowledge of the science and research taking place sheds light on what direction studies are taking and how they can be more universally impactful.

Knee Pain

Overview of Knee Pain

Knee pain happens when there is an issue in or around the joints and ligaments of the area. This is one condition that affects people of all ages, from all walks of life.

Common causes of long-term persistent knee pain include the following:

- Previous injury or tear
- Swelling or inflammation
- Arthritis or degenerative disease

For people with knee pain, they find out quickly that it is often persistent. The knee is one area of the body that can be affected so widely. Patients can struggle for many years, while they avoid surgery and work to find a comfortable option for their chronic pain.

Signs and Symptoms

Knee pain can be very different for patients with different health conditions and histories. Infection and inflammation will cause swelling over the entire knee. Other injuries might be more of a sharp pain in one specific area.

Location and severity of knee pain differs depending on factors such as these:

- Type of pain (sharp or dull)
- Severity of injury
- Quickness of onset

When the knee joint is weakened, symptoms can escalate quite quickly from a dull ache to severely limited mobility.

These are some of the most common symptoms for which patients seek health care:

- Shaking or unstable knee
- Inability to walk up or down stairs without pain
- Knee locking
- Popping or cracking sounds
- Swelling, redness, and tenderness of the area
- Favoring the other leg or limping
- Difficulty bending or straightening the knee.

Knee pain is so common because, as with all joints, there is a lot going on in a little area. Ligaments and tendons, when damaged, cause inflammation and problems in the rest of the knee. As well, previous injuries might not heal properly, depending on the medical care that the patient received.

Anatomy

The main function of the knee is to bend the leg to move the body (through walking). Much stress is put on this joint, as it bends, twists, and rotates throughout the day. The knee joint itself has three bones with many ligaments, tendons, and cartilage intertwined.

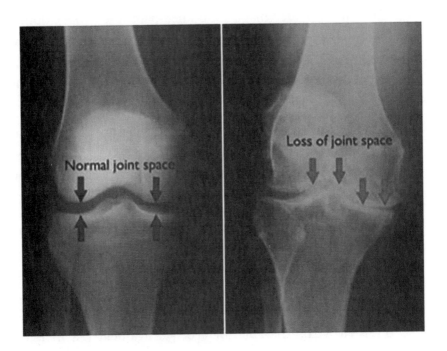

Risk Factors and Complications

Knee pain comes with its own set of risk factors and complications. As it is such an overused and complicated joint, there is much potential for small injuries to become complicated. These are the top three risk factors that can seriously impact the outcome of a knee condition.

1. **Excess Weight:** Causes stress on the knee joint
2. **Repetitive Movement:** Sports like skiing or jobs like floor installing can require the knees to move, twist, and strain

repetitively in the same way. Over time, this leads to serious problems.

3. **Smoking:** Patients who smoke have a higher risk for knee pain caused by arthritis.

Diagnosis and Testing

By a health-care provider diagnosing knee pain, the proper options for healing can be made available to a patient. For someone suffering through knee pain, this can be overwhelming and sometimes painful. It is however, necessary. The sooner you have a diagnosis and the proper testing done, the sooner you can find a solution that works.

The most common problems with knees fit into three separate categories: injuries, mechanical issues, and arthritis. Each of these is treated and tested differently, and each encompasses specific conditions with their own set of factors.

1. **Knee Injuries:** Happen when outside trauma affects knee function
   a. **Fractures:** Any of the three bones of the knee joint can be broken. People with weakened bone structure might experience this with very little impact.
   b. **Torn ACL:** The anterior cruciate ligament (ACL) is one of four ligaments connecting the knee to the shin. Often athletes and other people who are involved in overtly physical pursuits will experience this injury.
   c. **Torn Meniscus:** The meniscus is an area of cartilage that acts as a shock absorber between the thigh bone and shin bone. It is usually torn when the knee is twisted while bearing weight.
   d. **Tendinitis:** Tendinitis occurs when one or more tendons becomes irritated and inflamed, often due to overuse. The

patellar tendon attaches the quadriceps muscle to the front of the shinbone and is prone to irritation, especially in activities that involve jumping.

2. **Mechanical Problems:** Happen when there is an anatomical problem that affects knee pain
   a. **Dislocated Kneecap:** When the bone on the knee cap slips out of place.
   b. **Loose Debris:** Sometimes pieces of bone or cartilage break off and float around in the knee joint.
   c. **Hip or Foot Pain:** Pain in the hips or feet can change the way a person walks, and cause undue stress on the knee.
3. **Arthritis:** There are more than one hundred types of arthritis, most of which cause the cartilage in the joints to degenerate.

When medical treatment is sought out, the first step is in determining what the problem is. A series of tests to determine that exact nature of the condition may be pursued.

These are some of the tests that will help medical professionals discover what is going on in your knee:

- **X-ray:** Checking for fractures, degeneration, and arthritis
- **MRI:** Checking for tendon, muscle, and ligament issues
- **Blood Tests:** Checking for inflammation and gout

When to Seek Help

Often, people who have knee pain, especially when it is recurring, will suffer through it in silence, rather than seek help. There are circumstances, however, where it is not recommended to try to take care of it on your own.

It is recommended to seek help under any of the following circumstances:

1. Drastic increase in pain level
2. Inability to bend knee
3. Any sign of deformity
4. Infection/redness of the knee along with fever
5. Inability to walk or put weight on your knee

Treatment Options/Surgeries

In order to treat knee pain, there are several different options, depending on the cause and condition. In some cases, prescription medication can reduce pain, but it is also highly addictive. Surgery and knee replacements are common, but so is the increase of failed knee surgeries, where patients continue to suffer. Often, despite multiple surgeries, the patient sees little to no improvement.

Physical therapy is also used to improve knee pain, and provided the underlying condition is managed, these movements and exercises can help improve mobility and reduce pain and inflammation.

Other options that are used to treat knee pain include steroid injections (which if overused, cause degeneration of the joint), acupuncture (especially for patients with arthritis), and health supplements (for autoimmune-related inflammation).

Long-Term Outlook

The long-term outlook for knee pain, even with surgery and physical therapy is not a positive one. The problem is that the knees are the most-used joint in the body. It is difficult to allow an injury or condition time to heal, without causing major difficulty and inconvenience to the patient. It is next to impossible to live a healthy and productive life with knee pain because, over time, it will get worse.

Why Stem Cell Therapy

Stem cell therapy is a minimally invasive procedure for people suffering from knee pain. Knee pain is one of the most common reasons people seek stem cell therapy as an alternative to surgery. Although each patient will experience different results, many patients find long-term relief from the regenerative properties of stem cell therapy. Research has shown positive outcomes and improvement in the condition of cartilage and tendons. As the stem cells work with the body's natural healing ability, repair and regeneration of the knee joint occurs.

Jean's Story

"As a professional golfer for years, I was no stranger to knee pain. At the height of my career, I toured with the LPGA (Ladies Professional Golf Association) and was in the top ten for most of the season. As I climbed the ranks, my short game improved, and I thought this might be my year.

"I was one of the oldest women on the tour and felt like I had something to prove. It was now or never, and I wanted to retire to some golf club as a pro with something to show. It's funny how our memory works because I cannot recall any of that last game I played.

"All I remember is the searing pain as I tore the ligaments in my knee. And then, afterward, the doctors saying I would need to rest it for some months. All I knew is I was out for the rest of the season. It might as well have been forever.

"Determined to get back, I followed all the doctor's orders, but the pain persisted. Eventually, they tried surgery, and I remember

sitting in recovery thinking, "Okay, this is it; I get my life back now. But I didn't. Not yet, anyway.

"Apparently, I am one of the minority who gets worse after surgery—scar-tissue buildup, inflammation, and what I called a constant ache. When I walked, it got worse; forget about golf, I was done.

"Everyone always asks why I didn't fall into depression. Well, it is because I threw myself into finding another option. Even if I couldn't go pro again (I had given up that dream), I didn't have to give up on life.

"One of my friends introduced me to stem cell therapy, after talking about her mother and an unrelated issue. When I looked into it, I knew it would be the answer. It was my "aha" moment, and I had a really good feeling about it.

"The more I looked into it, the sooner I wanted to get it done; and now that I have gotten both knees done, I feel so positive about the future. With my first knee, it had been injured for so long, I was always babying it, which led me to the problem with my second knee.

"But then, things started to improve. The tightness and aching went away, and I had more mobility and I could finally be active again. It made me realize how important it was for me to be an athlete; to be involved in sport again is something that goes hand in hand with my health."

Stem Cell Therapy for Knee Joint Pain

As the science behind stem cell therapy continues to be researched, more specific studies are looking at how stem cells work in targeted ways. For knee-joint pain, *The Journal of Bone and Joint Surgery* completed:

> The first randomized, double-blind, controlled study to evaluate the safety, regenerative effects, and clinical outcomes of human mesenchymal stem cells delivered by intra-articular injection into the human knee. The results demonstrated that high doses of allogeneic mesenchymal stem cells can be safely delivered in a concentrated manner to an enclosed space (knee-joint capsule) without abnormal tissue formation.

Although more research is needed, this and other research is making clear the safety and efficacy of stem cell treatment in a broad range of issues. For knee pain, the ability of the stem cells to mitigate the damage to the meniscal tissue of the knee joint is worth further investigation. As well, the possibility of positive changes and reduced future damage shows the adaptability of stem cell therapy.

Research Articles

There are many research articles related to stem cell therapy for knee pain, including the following:

1. Mesenchymal stem cell therapy for knee osteoarthritis: Five-years follow-up of three patients
2. Restoration of a large osteochondral defect of the knee using a composite of umbilical cord blood-derived mesenchymal stem cells and hyaluronic acid hydrogel: A case report with a five-year follow-up

3. Adult Human Mesenchymal Stem Cells Delivered via Intra-Articular Injection to the Knee Following Partial Medial Meniscectomy

You can find PDFs of the articles on my website www.regenhealthmed.com under patient resources.

Hip Pain

What Is Hip Pain?

The hip is probably the most-used joint in the body for most people, and it can also be a place of great pain. Physically, it is comprised of a ball and socket that attaches the leg to the torso. Almost every movement we make involves the hip joint, and pain in this area becomes more and more frequent with age.

The combination of how frequently people use their legs and how the socket of the hip itself is situated creates a high possibility of a problem in the area. The socket of the hip is part of the pelvic bone. In this area, the spinal cord and many nerve endings are moving through a relatively small space. As well, there are ligaments, tendons, and connective tissue working to bend and step, sit and stand.

People who suffer with hip pain all have one thing in common: hip pain generally gets worse over time. Although there are many different problems and conditions associated with hip pain, they all result in a deterioration in overall well-being.

Common Causes of Hip Pain:

- Trauma or injury
- Inflammation
- Bone disease

- Arthritis
- Fibromyalgia
- Sciatica or other nerve pain
- Fracture or dislocation
- Back problems
- Autoimmune disease
- Bacterial infections

Signs and Symptoms

With hip pain, the onset and symptoms will vary from patient to patient. Since it is such a complex joint with lots of interconnecting systems, it can be easy to mistake some symptoms for another problem. As well, it can be difficult to pinpoint exactly where the problem is.

The most common symptoms of hip pain include these:

- Difficulty or stiffness when bending or twisting
- Feeling worse after exercise
- Cracking or popping during movement
- Arthritis, aches, or joint problems
- Sudden impact or other injury
- Nerve problems
- Weakness in legs or limping

Anatomy

Hip pain is sometimes difficult to diagnose due to the multiple body systems and components in the area:

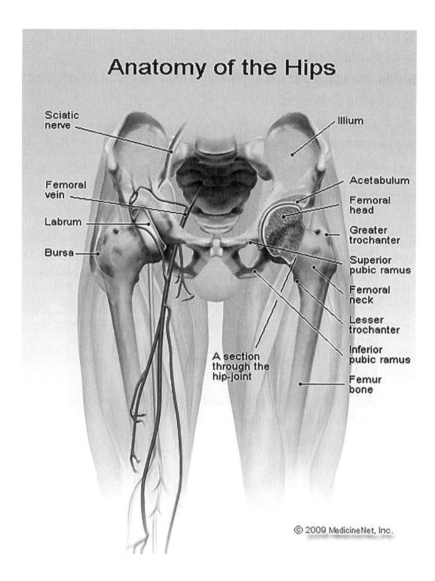

Anatomy of the Hips

Sciatic nerve

Illium

Femoral vein

Acetabulum

Femoral head

Labrum

Greater trochanter

Bursa

Superior pubic ramus

Femoral neck

Lesser trochanter

A section through the hip-joint

Inferior pubic ramus

Femur bone

© 2009 MedicineNet, Inc.

Diagnosis and Testing

For patients with hip pain, the first step to diagnosis is often a visit to an emergency room. Hip pain can be sudden and unexpected, as in accidents or injuries. Other times, it is a part of aging, and the condition worsens over time.

Either way, the doctor will start with a physical examination to determine the location and type of pain, the movement capabilities, and family history of the patient. From there, specific tests are requisitioned to investigate the problem more closely.

Routine blood work and an X-ray are the first tests completed. The exact location of the pain is important to determine before any treatment options are considered. From there, a MRI or bone scan can be completed to outline, more exactly, the area where the joint is damaged, and check for inflammation.

Risk Factors

Hip pain, as we have seen, does not have one cause, but most people with hip pain share similar risk factors. These are some of the contributing factors to the immune system attacking the body:

- **Obesity:** An increase in weight can cause or worsen hip pain putting more stress on the joints and other body systems.
- **Genetics:** Genetic factors can increase certain problems that cause hip pain.
- **Weak Bones:** Osteoporosis and other bone-weakening disorders can increase the likelihood of hip problems.

When to Seek Help

For patients with hip pain, the severity of their discomfort often drives them to seek medical help quite suddenly. If an accident or possible break occurs, it is important to have a doctor or surgeon assess your condition.

In situations with gradual or long-term hip pain, it is not necessarily as clear when additional treatment might be required. When a patient has known hip pain and then experiences a quick change in the condition, it is important to find the cause. Sudden loss of movement, increase in pain, or loss of bladder or other functions can be a signal something more serious is going on.

Treatment Options/Surgeries

Treatment options for hip pain usually depend on a three-pronged approach, specially suited to both the condition and the individual's health needs.

1. **Basic:** Over-the-counter pain medication, ice and heat treatment, physiotherapy, prescription medicine, rest
2. **Advanced:** Injections, long-term medication, lifestyle or activity change
3. **Severe:** Hip replacement

Why Stem Cell Therapy

Many of the symptoms and causes of hip pain are associated with the body's aging. Stem cell therapy provides the regeneration and repair the joint needs to regain normal function. Patients are beginning to hear about regenerative medicine as an option to reduce symptoms of hip pain.

This is especially the case for hip pain caused by inflammation-related issues. The anti-inflammatory properties of stem cells are bringing relief to patients with arthritis and other autoimmune issues.

Frank's Story

"When my hip started bugging me, I denied it for a while and made it out to be not as bad as it was. I couldn't fool everyone though, and my wife knew better. She convinced me that I needed to see a doctor and really find out what the problem was. The doctor was surprised I had not been in sooner, as I had significant inflammation and was eventually diagnosed with arthritis.

"Of course, it doesn't end there; as I wasn't responding to treatment, the doctors kept looking for what they might be missing. For a while, it felt like everything was getting worse—the pain, the medical treatment, my ability to walk.

"When my wife suggested a cane, I got angry. I wasn't angry with her; I just didn't want to let go, and having a cane felt like I had one foot in the grave. With a cane, I didn't want to go anywhere. My friends are the kind of guys to relentlessly mock one of our buddies for a cane, for getting older. I would have done the same to any of them. But it bugged me a lot, probably because it was the truth.

"One day, when one of my wife's friends was visiting, she mentioned stem cell therapy. Right away, for some reason, I just knew it would work out. She referred me to her doctor, and at the first appointment, all my questions were answered.

"After I received stem cell therapy, my hip pain became less and less severe. I began walking without a cane and didn't have a pained expression on my face every time I moved. It amazes me how quick and easy the procedure was for me to end up with these results. It is way beyond anything I could have expected.

"Before my hip problems, I had never heard of stem cell therapy, but now it is something I hear about quite a bit. Now almost everyone knows someone who has had the procedure, and I haven't heard a bad story yet. I am glad it is becoming more common because I sure would have liked to have had it offered as one of my first options, instead of struggling for so long like I did."

Stem Cells in the Treatment of Hip Pain

Science and research into stem cells for hip pain is confirming the stories and research of clinical trials; and a reduction in symptoms and improvement of quality of life is the common outcome.

One study in the *Journal of Hip Preservation Surgery,* showed that shortly after receiving stem cell therapy, a significant improvement in hip function was experienced. As well, "The reparative effect, which is fully maintained over time, proved to be free of major complications or side effects during the prolonged follow-up period. Moreover, the radiographic scores of the hip joint(s), assessed on a time period ranging from seven to thirty months after cell infusion, clearly demonstrate a halt in the progression of osteoarthritis."

These positive results are spurring more study into regenerative properties of stem cells. As science proves the stem cells repair and improve function on joints like the hip, the procedure will become more well-known and recommended.

Shoulder Pain

Overview of Shoulder Pain

Shoulder pain is one condition that most people experience at one time or another. The pain can come from the shoulder or any of the muscles, ligaments, or tendons connected to the area. If the pain gets worse with movement of the shoulder, it is usually an issue with the joint.

Rotator cuff tears are one of the most common conditions for chronic shoulder pain. This small tendon is easily torn and has difficulty regenerating, especially with age and continued wear and tear.

In attempting to improve pain and other symptoms of shoulder pain, the following treatments are common:

- Surgical repair
- Physical therapy
- Massage
- Steroid injections
- Painkillers

Chronic shoulder pain is often a decades-long struggle for many people. Since the shoulder is a joint that is used for almost every activity, it can be difficult to get the time to rest and repair any damage. As well, many parts are working together, so there is a lot more that can go wrong.

Common Causes of Shoulder Pain

The shoulder is similar to the knee in that it is a complex joint that is used frequently. Often, causes of shoulder pain can be mitigated by monitoring the type of actions and movements being used.

That being said, almost all shoulder problems fit into one of four categories of cause:

1. **Broken Bone:** A fracture has occurred in one of the shoulder bones.
2. **Tendon Issues:** Inflammation, tendonitis, or a tear can all cause shoulder pain.
3. **Arthritis:** Degeneration of the tissue in the joint
4. **Instability:** Muscular issues

Signs and Symptoms

Shoulder pain can be gradual or sudden, depending on the cause and severity of the issue. An immediate accident or injury is often the first sign of shoulder pain. In other cases, it can start as a dull ache or pain from an unknown origin.

Some symptoms are surprising, as they do not even come from the shoulder. Others are more obvious. Checking the type and duration of symptoms… helps determine possible healing solutions.

In the shoulder area, pain symptoms can vary considerably, although these are some of the most common experiences:

- Redness, swelling, or bruising
- Inability to raise arm above head
- Stabbing or burning sensation in your shoulder
- Shooting pain from shoulder to elbow and beyond
- Dull ache during repetitive movement

Anatomy

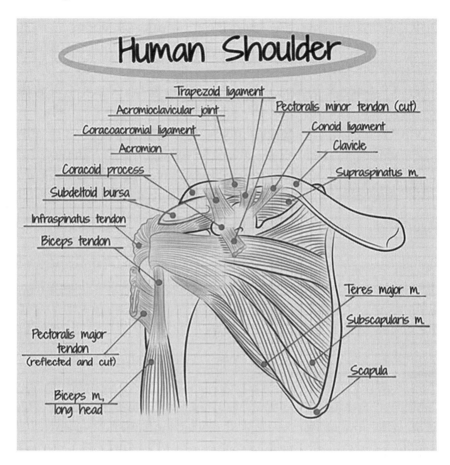

Diagnosis and Testing

Shoulder pain requires an in-depth physical examination to check range of movement, physical abnormalities or deformities, and muscle weakness. From there, the health-care team can determine what further actions are required.

In almost every situation, further testing is required to see what is happening inside the shoulder joint to pinpoint the problem.

The most frequent tests for shoulder pain include the following:

1. **X-ray:** To check whether there are any broken bones
2. **MRI and Ultrasound:** To check for tissue and ligament damage or abnormalities
3. **CT Scan:** Provides a digital overview of an X-ray to view the shoulder bones
4. **Arthroscopy:** A surgical procedure where a camera is inserted in the shoulder to look more closely at soft tissue and to check for issues the other tests might have missed. During this procedure, small repairs can often be made, if necessary.

When to Seek Help

Shoulder pain is also associated with heart attack. If you experience sudden shoulder or arm pain on your left side, especially alongside a tightness in the chest, light-headedness, or shortness of breath, seek immediate medical help.

Treatment Options/Surgeries

Aside from arthroscopy, which was described above, there are a few different treatment options and surgeries available to patients with shoulder pain. Depending on the situation and severity, one or more of these might be used to regain mobility and reduce pain.

1. **Physical Therapy:** Trying different movements and rest to minimize stress on the joint can help improve the shoulder pain.
2. **Medication:** Used to reduce inflammation and manage pain. Caution is advised, as it can be easy to do more damage to the shoulder when the area is numbed by painkillers.
3. **Surgery:** For more serious injuries, surgery might be required to repair tissue or replace the shoulder joint entirely.

Long-Term Outlook

For many patients with shoulder pain, the long-term outlook is very promising. Although, like the knee, there are many complexities in the shoulder, there is also less stress put on it so that rest and healing are more feasible. The shoulder can be immobile quite naturally.

In some patients, often after surgery or steroid injections, there might be chronic pain and problems that keep reappearing.

Why Stem Cell Therapy

For me, when people ask why they should consider stem cell therapy to treat their shoulder pain, I always tell them to review the many comments offered by patients. I refer them to the many research, clinical trials, and stories like Helen's story, below. When people experience the healing, they are happy to share their experiences.

Stem cell therapy offers a regenerative option that is unlike anything else the medical system has. It is noninvasive and will not exacerbate the problem. The natural healing ability of your body is worn down over time, and stem cell therapy is a boost to that system. For many patients, the reduction in pain is only one of the many benefits they see.

Helen's Story

"When I went for stem cell therapy, it was just the next thing in a long list of things I tried. By that time, it was just a process, I had no expectation of hope or help. My shoulder pain numbed my life, and I didn't see anything that would fix it.

"My shoulder had hurt on and off for as long as I can remember. Then I went bowling with some friends and hurt myself. I don't even know how I did it, we were just being silly. It was my turn, and I twisted funny and I felt a searing burning sensation. Since then, I couldn't lift my arm above my head.

"Doctors said it was my rotator cuff and sent me to a chiropractor. The chiropractor said it would take time, and I thought I was seeing minor improvement. Until I wasn't. Then I tried steroid injections, and that worked for a while.

"When the pain came back, I just changed how I lived. I stopped going out; I couldn't put things away up high or properly take care of my apartment. The pain and numbness was starting to spread down my arm and into my hand. As well, I was wearing out my other arm with overuse.

"Something had to give, but I just kept going to doctors who had no suggestions. So when I saw an ad for stem cell therapy that recommended use for shoulder pain, I figured I had tried everything else, why not one more thing.

"The fact is stem cell therapy has helped so much more than my shoulder. Every week that went by, I started feeling better and better. My movement is better, and I can use my arm just the way I used to."

Stem Cells for Shoulder Pain

Even with improved surgical and medical treatment, rotator cuff injuries are still seen as an ongoing, chronic pain for many patients. The tendons, bones, ligaments, and muscles are under constant stress, so healing strategies must be carefully construed. Research is showing the successful application of stem cells for shoulder pain.

A study about stem cell therapy with shoulder pain patients showed:

> Fourteen patients with a complete tear of the rotator cuff that was repaired in a trans osseous fashion through a mini-incision augmenting the suture with mononuclear stem cells from iliac crest bone-marrow aspirate. At twelve months, twelve of the fourteen tears had healed according to clinical and magnetic resonance imaging results.

The potential for stem cell therapy in regeneration and healing in joint and muscle issues in the shoulder and surrounding area is seen to be overwhelmingly positive. By reducing inflammation and directing the cells right at the source of the issue, there are no negative side effects, and the majority of patients experience significant improvement.

Rheumatoid Arthritis/Osteoarthritis

Overview of Arthritis

Arthritis occurs when there is inflammation in one or multiple joints. The main symptoms are stiffness and pain that worsens as the condition carries on. There are more than one hundred known causes of arthritis. The swelling leads to a reduced range of movement and limited mobility for patients suffering from arthritis.

These are the two most frequently diagnosed types of arthritis:

Osteoarthritis (OA)

- Normal wear and tear and degeneration are the most common causes of OA.
- Infection or injury can worsen OA as it speeds up the natural breakdown of cartilage in the joints.
- People with a genetic connection to this disease through family history are more likely to see symptoms.

Rheumatoid Arthritis (RA)

- RA is an autoimmune disorder.
- As the disease progresses, the immune system attacks and destroys both the bone and cartilage inside the joint.
- If left untreated, RA can lead to permanent deformity and disability.

Current treatment involves monitoring the condition and prescribing medication. Research is showing continued improvement for patients who try stem cell therapy to improve arthritis.

Signs and Symptoms

For simplicity sake, we will separate rheumatoid arthritis and osteoarthritis to make it easy for readers to see what applies to their personal situation.

Rheumatoid arthritis sufferers experience these symptoms:

- Fatigue
- Pain and tenderness
- Swelling and redness or warmth
- Joint stiffness
- Reduced range of motion

Osteoarthritis sufferers experience these symptoms:

- Pain during movement
- Loss of flexibility
- Joint stiffness or tenderness
- Bone-on-bone feeling

Anatomy

NORMAL AND ARTHRITIC JOINTS

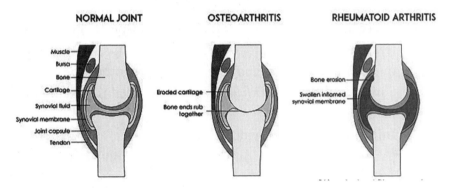

Risk Factors and Complications

For both types of arthritis, the risk factors and complications are similar. Long-term inflammation and degeneration of the joints leads to loss of movement and increase in chronic pain.

Risk factors that increase likelihood of arthritis include the following:

1. **Age:** The older a person is, the higher the risk.
2. **Gender:** Females are more likely to have arthritis than males.
3. **Injury:** Injury or repeated stress to the area
4. **Genetic factors**

When to Seek Help

If you have pain or stiffness in any part of your body that will not go away, it is important to get advice from a medical professional.

Treatment Options/Surgeries

When you are diagnosed with arthritis, you and your doctor should come up with a treatment plan that suits your symptoms and conditions. Often a combination of medication, lifestyle changes, and possibly even surgery are the only options given to patients to manage their arthritis.

1. **Exercise and Diet:** Two important aspects of arthritis treatment. Many doctors do not discuss this, as they focus on the test results and medication or other treatments. Eating healthy and staying active are crucial in regenerating deteriorating joints.
2. **Injections:** These provide a short-term relief of pain, so the patient can participate in physical therapy and resume daily activities.
3. **Fluid Removal (arthrocentesis):** Relieves pressure and joint pain caused by fluid buildup. Once fluid is removed, it is often sent for testing.
4. **Medication:** Different conditions will be treated with different medications, including prescription opioids. As well, over-the-counter medications such as ibuprofen might provide relief.
5. **Surgery:** From microscopic surgery to total-joint replacement, the end result for some arthritis patients is surgery to help get some relief from the pain.

Long-Term Outlook

Osteoarthritis gets worse over time, as the degeneration to the joint does not stop. The pain, stiffness, and lack of movement eventually prevent people from having the quality of life they previously experienced. Most people believe a joint replacement surgery is the only long-term option.

For patients with rheumatoid arthritis, there seem to be more options. Since it is an inflammatory issue, the underlying condition can be found and improved. At the same time, inflammation and autoimmune issues are complex unto themselves, and it is often difficult to ascertain the exact cause.

Why Stem Cell Therapy

For both osteoarthritis and rheumatoid arthritis, stem cell therapy encourages regeneration of the joint. It also reduces inflammation, which is especially beneficial for rheumatoid arthritis patients, since arthritis causes severe pain and disability. The long-term relief and improvement of symptoms being seen in research and through patients' experiences are showing very positive results.

Bill's Story

"I've been on meds for severe rheumatoid arthritis for so many years I lost count. It was a daily struggle and what felt like constant pain. After a lifetime in an active job, being able to do basically what I wanted, I felt like the end was near.

"As the months went on with no end in sight, I cried at night when my wife was sleeping because there was no rest for me. It was agony to try to get dressed, and my one leg was always dragging; I just had no strength in it.

"All the pain and swelling was becoming just too much. My wife had to help me with everything, even getting out of my chair. My son told me about stem cell therapy after taking a holiday in Panama, where he met more than one person who had traveled there specifically for that reason. He said it is quite common for people to travel, but that I could get the therapy right near by.

"When I received the stem cell therapy, I was dubious. Over the weeks after, though, I noticed little things. First, it was at night. I was sleeping so much better. The first time I woke up from a really good sleep, I was a bit stunned. I had forgotten how it felt to sleep hard, without tossing and turning in pain all night.

"Then I got up out of my chair, and my wife just looked at me. Her face was filled with joy as she realized I was regaining my freedom. It was freedom for her as well, as so much of her time was taken up in caring for me.

"Now my quality of life has gone way up. I continue to see little improvements. Even my doctors could not deny the difference in my condition."

Stem Cell Treatment for Patients with Arthritis

The research is beginning to catch up to the experiences of patients, such as the positive results seen in a study on Spondyloarthritis (SpA):

> . . . stem cells of hematopoietic origin, MSCs have also caught the attention of researchers. For instance, Huang et al [76] have investigated the inhibitory effects of human umbilical cord derived MSCs (hUCMSCs) on peripheral blood T cells from

patients with SpA in vivo in search of their therapeutic potential. It was found that co-culturing of peripheral blood mononuclear cells (PBMNC) with hUCMSCs significantly reduced IL-17 production from peripheral blood T cells, suggesting that MSCs may be a good candidate for the treatment of SpA.

Spondyloarthritis (SpA) is the name for the multiple, interrelated types of inflammatory arthritis including these:

- Ankylosing spondylitis (AS)
- Psoriatic arthritis
- Reactive arthritis
- Rheumatoid arthritis (RA)

This study covers the uses of stem cell therapy for arthritis and the potential complications that can arise. The potential for future therapies and benefits to those who experience inflammatory arthritis is in continued research using umbilical cord stem cells.

Research Articles

There are many research articles related to stem cell therapy for arthritis including the following:

1. Mesenchymal stem cells for cartilage repair in osteoarthritis
2. Stem cell research on arthritis
3. The potential role of adult stem cells in the management of rheumatic diseases

You can find the PDF article on my website www.regenhealthmed.com under patient resources.

Parkinson's Disease

Overview of Parkinson's Disease

Parkinson's disease is a degeneration of the nervous system caused by death of neurotransmitters in certain areas of the brain.

These are some of the most common symptoms experienced by those suffering from Parkinson's disease:

- Tremors
- Stiff muscles
- Loss of speech
- Loss of control of limbs
- Choking, difficulty swallowing, and drooling
- Bladder dysfunction
- Sleep disorders

Currently the medical treatment for Parkinson's simply addresses the symptoms, trying to bring some semblance of comfort to patients. But it does nothing to improve the underlying cause of the disease.

Common Causes

In Parkinson's patients, the cells of the nervous system die off. Although currently there is not one known cause of Parkinson's disease, there are several factors that are attributed with the disease.

These are some of the known factors that increase the likelihood of contracting Parkinson's:

- Genetic mutations
- Exposure to toxins
- Changes in brain cell composition
- Aged sixty or older
- Male gender has a higher rate of the disease

Anatomy

Parkinson's disease is caused by the gradual death of neurons in the brain, especially in the region of the substantia nigra (SN). This area regulates dopamine release. As the disease progresses, the loss of dopamine inhibits motor function, and movements become more and more uncontrollable.

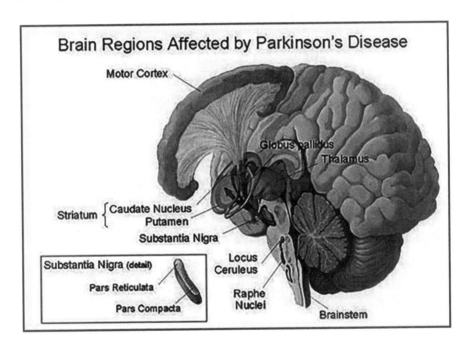

Complications

As Parkinson's develops and further degeneration occurs, the symptoms of the disease can begin to cause a disruption to quality of life. In this way, the medical team ends up treating each symptom to alleviate some of the pain and discomfort, even though there is no real improvement being made.

Reducing just one of the following complications allows the patient to regain some semblance of freedom:

- **Cognitive Problems (Dementia):** This is associated with the degenerated brain cells, and Parkinson's patients often see a deterioration in their ability to perform simple mental tasks. Their memory and ability to reason is also, often, affected.
- **Loss of Bladder and Bowel Control:** Patients often experience constipation and an inability to urinate.
- **Pain and Fatigue:** Many people with Parkinson's disease experience pain in either one area or throughout their bodies. It is also common for them to lack energy and feel an overall weakness.
- **Problems Swallowing:** As the disease progresses, people may experience difficulty swallowing. Often, saliva accumulates because of an inability to swallow, which leads to excessive drooling.

Diagnosis and Testing

Currently, there is no specific test to determine Parkinson's disease. A neurologist will diagnose a patient based on medical history, symptoms, and other factors. Often, it takes time to determine that Parkinson's disease is the problem as doctors rule out other issues first.

There might be blood and other tests to verify the condition is not something else before the doctor can confirm. As well, there is a medication that can be prescribed if Parkinson's is suspected. The medication usually helps patients with Parkinson's, so if someone sees results with this medication, the results are often used to provide confirmation of diagnosis.

When to Seek Help

If you are experiencing symptoms associated with Parkinson's disease, consult a doctor. It is important to get diagnosed to assess your condition and to rule out any other complications.

Treatment Options/Surgeries

There is no cure for Parkinson's disease, though prescription medication, including cannabis, provides patients with relief from symptoms and an improved quality of life. In some cases, a physical and speech therapist will offer help with exercises.

Since a loss of dopamine is a result of Parkinson's disease, medications that mimic or convert to dopamine are often very beneficial in reducing tremors and other symptoms. As the disease progresses, the medication can become less effective and might have to be changed or used in conjunction with another prescription.

For patients with advanced Parkinson's, surgery in the form of deep brain stimulation (DBS) is one treatment option. During this procedure, electrodes are implanted inside the brain and then a generator is implanted at the collarbone to send electrical impulses to the electrodes. Although invasive, this surgical procedure reduces tremors and involuntary movements in patients whose medication is no longer working adequately.

Long-Term Outlook

Parkinson's disease is a chronic illness that worsens over time. The physical limitations of the disease can lead to emotional and mental issues as the patient struggles to cope with loss of bodily functions. Medications lose efficacy over time, and it can be difficult to continually change prescriptions and adapt to new side effects.

Why Stem Cell Therapy

The regenerative properties of stem cell therapy are having a positive effect on Parkinson's patients. Research showing stem cells creating dopamine-producing cells is promising. Although it is a new therapy for a serious disease, more and more patients are regaining control of their health using stem cell therapy.

Stem Cell Therapy for Parkinson's

Recent research is showing the length of time stem cells remain active in the body is affecting improvement in Parkinson's patients. Scientists are looking at how stem cell therapy is working in patients over a specific time period.

"Researchers have pursued the idea that pluripotent stem cells, which can form any cell type in the body, could replace dead dopamine-making neurons in people with Parkinson's, and thus potentially halt or even reverse disease progression."

The results in nonhuman trials are connecting stem cell therapy to new and improved connections in brain cells and body function.

Research

There are many research articles related to stem cell therapy for Parkinson's, including the following:

Hematopoietic stem and progenitor cells in the treatment of severe autoimmune diseases

You can find the PDF article on my website www.regenhealthmed.com under patient resources.

Autoimmune Diseases

What Is Autoimmune Disease?

Autoimmune disease is what happens when the immune system attacks the body's own systems. Depending on the region and type of attack, different symptoms present themselves. There are more than 150 different autoimmune diseases, many of which we discuss in this book.

The individual aspects of a person's body makeup, diet, and lifestyle all contribute to the autoimmune condition. Whatever the cause, the immune system affects the function of different systems in the body, creating or compounding health problems.

The medical system practice is to treat the symptoms, as there are no cures for many of these diseases. Stem cell therapy acts to balance the regenerative abilities of the body, reducing inflammation and encouraging healing.

Common Autoimmune Diseases

Type 1 diabetes	Rheumatoid arthritis (RA)
Psoriasis/psoriatic arthritis	Multiple sclerosis (MS)
Lupus	Inflammatory bowel disease
Addison's disease	Graves' disease
Sjögren's syndrome	Hashimoto's thyroiditis
Myasthenia gravis	Vasculitis
Pernicious anemia	Celiac disease
Crohn's disease	Alopecia
Endometriosis	Ulcerative colitis
Fibromyalgia	and many more . . .

Signs and Symptoms

Although each individual autoimmune disease has its own systems being affected with corresponding symptoms, the diseases often overlap. That being said, there are some symptoms that are common among most autoimmune diseases.

Although each patient will react to the autoimmune issue differently, most of the following symptoms are some of the first signs of trouble patients will bring up to their doctors:

- Abdominal pain or digestive issues
- Low energy, feeling sluggish
- Swollen glands, fever
- Feeling worse after exercise
- Lack of focus, having a hard time paying attention
- Difficulty remembering things or learning new things
- Swollen or tightness in throat
- Dry hair and skin
- Trouble with speech, snoring, and mouth problems
- Arthritis, aches, or joint problems
- Nerve problems like carpal tunnel syndrome

Anatomy

Autoimmune diseases can affect so many different parts of the body, as can be seen below.

Depending on the type of autoimmune disease, a more precise look at the specific anatomy being affected is required. For example, a patient with Hashimoto's thyroiditis would want to understand the thyroid anatomy.

Diagnosis and Testing

There is no one test for autoimmune disease, and it is often one of the most difficult to determine as so many of the symptoms seem unrelated or potentially caused by something with a simpler explanation. Testing and diagnosis usually start with specific symptoms and then expand, based on what is found.

For example, a patient who is tired all the time and can no longer seem to concentrate might visit a doctor. From there, after a physical exam, the doctor might discover an enlarged thyroid, and then blood work and other tests will be done to confirm whether it is an autoimmune issue.

The same thing happens for other conditions, and the autoimmune diagnosis usually comes after significant testing is done for individual symptoms.

Risk Factors

Autoimmune diseases do not have one cause, but they do all share similar risk factors. These are some of the contributing factors to the immune system attacking the body:

- **Obesity:** When the body is overweight, there is a higher risk of autoimmune disease due, in part, to fat cells encouraging inflammation, as well as the weight putting more stress on the joints and other body systems.
- **Genetics:** Many autoimmune conditions have genetic factors, which are not fully understood. Certain diseases like lupus and multiple sclerosis have a genetic component; however, a family history does not guarantee a patient will contract the disease.
- **Smoking:** Research has found a correlation between smoking and autoimmune disease as smokers have a higher likelihood

of being diagnosed with rheumatoid arthritis, hypothyroid, and other conditions.

When to Seek Help

If you have previously not had any health issues and suddenly experience extreme fatigue, joint issues, or some of the other symptoms combined with weakness or loss of energy, do not overlook it. Autoimmune diseases are best treated early, and often, the first sign is a patient who is feeling that something about their health is different or not quite right.

Treatment Options/Surgeries

A treatment program for autoimmune disease usually incorporates a three-pronged approach, especially suited to both the condition and the individual's health needs:

1. **Symptom Relief:** First and foremost, the conditions of the disease are brought under control through medication and other therapies.

2. **Protecting Organs:** Medication and other treatment options are used to prevent the specific body systems from being destroyed.

3. **Suppressing the Immune System:** By suppressing the immune system, treatment can target how the autoimmune condition works to prevent it from spreading.

Why Stem Cell Therapy

Stem cell therapy is especially beneficial in autoimmune conditions because of the anti-inflammatory properties of stem cells. The other benefit is the ability for stem cells to regenerate and repair damaged tissue.

The noninvasive procedure can be used to target the exact area, specific to whichever part of the body the autoimmune disease is attacking.

Sal's Story

"Retirement was my golden apple, and I worked, often sixty hours a week, to get there. After my forty years of service, I got a big ceremony, a clock, and the jealousy of everyone in the office who still had years to go.

"After a few months, I took my wife on a cruise, and we began to plan life as a retired couple. It was our dream to get an RV and travel around the country to all of the national parks. We were going to sell our house to pay for it, and get a little condo on the oceanfront for the winters or when we didn't want to travel.

"The house was for sale, and we were shopping for RVs, planning our route, and keeping an eye out for the perfect condo. But for me, I was feeling worn out. Everything took a little extra energy. I felt sore and achy, and the doctors kept telling me I was fine, and it was just old age.

"Well, I didn't believe old age happened overnight, and I wanted some answers, but I was too tired to look. The symptoms began to build up, and eventually, we took the house off the market and just spent our time managing my health issues.

"My wife kept trying to get me to try different things, but I was fairly stubborn about it. Finally, she just took me to the consultation about stem cells without discussing it with me. And as usual, my wife was right.

"Having gone through stem cell therapy, I do not understand why it is not the go-to therapy for people with autoimmune. I mean, it just makes sense. The science behind it—their website can explain it better than I can—is so clearly fixing the problem because of how stem cells work.

"Put it this way, five weeks after the therapy, I felt like I was back to my old self again. In fact, my wife was so hopeful, she started looking at condos again, and I am just so happy to be awake and rejuvenated. It made me realize my health is the golden apple, not retirement."

Stem Cells in the Treatment of Autoimmune Disease

In specific research papers on the effects of autoimmune disease on stem cells, the regenerative properties of the therapies are showing very successful results. Human stem cells (HSCs) derived from umbilical cord blood are being studied.

The results are beginning to show that: "HSCs play a fundamental role in controlling chronic inflammation and immune regulation and are capable of regenerating immune cells. They are characterized by their ability to self-renew and also to differentiate into diverse types of blood cells."

The outlook for results with stem cell therapy on autoimmune disease is very promising as it addresses the inflammation that is a common symptom among all different conditions.

Research

There are many research articles related to stem cell therapy for autoimmune disease, including the following:

1. Hematopoietic stem and progenitor cells in the treatment of severe autoimmune diseases
2. Improvement of inflammatory bowel disease after allogeneic stem cell transplantation
3. Stem cells as potential targeted therapy for inflammatory bowel disease

You can find the PDFs of the articles on my website www.regenhealthmed.com under patient resources.

Cardiovascular Disease

Overview of Cardiovascular Disease

Also called *heart disease,* cardiovascular disease includes diseases that affect the heart and blood vessels. Degeneration, inflammation, and reduced function occur to offset the effects of the disease. Cardiovascular disease is the leading cause of death worldwide, according to the World Health Organization. One in every four women will die from cardiovascular disease.

These are some of the most commonly diagnosed cardiovascular diseases:

- Angina
- Hypertension
- Coronary artery disease
- Cardiomyopathy

Different factors like health, age, diet, and environment can increase risk for cardiovascular disease. Other than medication to reduce symptoms, surgery, including heart transplantation, has been the main medical treatment to date. Often risky or fatal, surgery only fixes the current problem and does not prevent it from returning.

Common Causes

Causes of cardiovascular disease are the same, across the board. High blood pressure and fatty deposits lining the blood vessels and arteries cause permanent damage to the heart muscle and function. The most obvious causes of cardiovascular disease are things that damage the heart.

In some cases, a virus, infection, or other condition damages the circulatory system. When this happens, the result is the same as above.

Signs and Symptoms

As with other conditions, symptoms vary from person to person. That being said, there are still common symptoms that most people who suffer from cardiovascular disease experience. Some of these include the following:

- Pressure in the chest
- Weakness and fatigue
- Pain in the arms, shoulder, jaw, or back
- Shortness of breath
- Feeling dizzy or light-headed

Anatomy

Seeing the image below sheds light on the severity of cardiovascular disease. As the heart struggles to pump, it is obvious that the symptoms will only increase as the disease progresses.

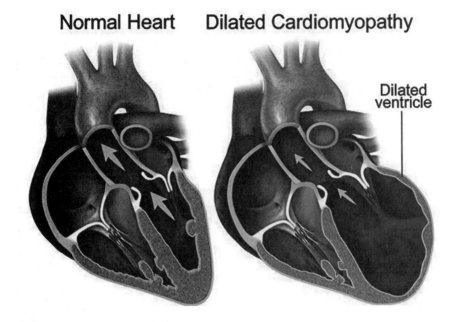

Normal Heart   Dilated Cardiomyopathy

Dilated ventricle

Diagnosis and Testing

A medical team performs various examinations and tests prior to diagnosis. Depending on your health, family history, and symptoms, the doctor will decide what further tests are needed.

Other than routine bloodwork, these are some of the other tests for cardiovascular disease:

- **Chest X-ray:** To provide an initial picture of what is going on inside.
- **Electrocardiogram (ECG):** Detects irregularities in the rhythm and structure of heart beats. This test is often done at rest, and then again, while active.
- **Echocardiogram:** A detailed image of the heart's structure and function.
- **Stress Test:** Checking how the heart responds to stress by increase heart rate under specific conditions.

Treatment Options

Cardiovascular disease, in all its forms, leads to offers of three treatment options provided by mainstream medical personnel. For many, they work in conjunction with one another to provide a whole-healing experience.

1. **Lifestyle Changes:** From what you eat to how often you sleep and how much physical activity you undertake, all these choices can affect heart health.
2. **Medication:** Doctors will prescribe medication to stop the damage of heart disease.
3. **Surgery:** Different surgeries to bypass or replace clogged arteries are common, but they are serious and take time to recover from.

Long-Term Outlook

Cardiovascular disease can have an extremely positive long-term outlook as people find healing options and choose to live a more heart-healthy life. So many people who are diagnosed with cardiovascular disease reverse their symptoms and recover their well-being.

On the other hand, there are other factors, like genetics, at play. There are times when an otherwise healthy individual drops dead of a heart attack with what seems like no warning.

Both examples are extreme cases on opposite ends of the spectrum. The point is that every patient is different, and every one of them needs to take into consideration their own personal health situation.

Why Stem Cell Therapy

For patients with cardiovascular disease, stem cell therapy offers a noninvasive way to promote healing and regeneration. Since heart health is connected to the entire body, this option, combined with lifestyle choices and a commitment to wellness, often can transform people's lives. Rather than relying on medications, with sometimes detrimental side effects, stem cell therapy is focused on using the body's natural ability to repair itself.

Lou's Story

"I had been warned about my heart problems for years. And for years, I took my medication, but did not change my lifestyle. I ate poorly and didn't take care of myself, and then I blamed myself for my health problems, and down I spiraled.

"Because I didn't have any family around, I didn't feel encouraged to improve myself in any way. I was always tired and depressed, and I lost my zeal for life. My friends started to be concerned when I stopped coming to our weekly card game. The truth was I was in bed before supper time, just exhausted.

"I also had a high level of anxiety all the time. It was like I was a ticking time bomb, and I didn't know how long my heart would last. It was really scary. When my doctor wanted to change my medication, I really began to wonder whether there was a better way.

"Once I looked into it, I thought stem cell therapy seemed too good to be true. So I made sure I got all my questions answered and looked at any possible risks. There were none that I could see, and the staff at the office and the doctors were so professional. For once, it felt like I was being heard.

> *"After the therapy, the way I put it is that I began to feel normal again. My shortness of breath and exhaustion were gone. I went back to playing cards and just getting out again. Sure, I still had to make those lifestyle changes I had been avoiding, but at least I had hope and I saw that it was possible for my body to heal."*

Umbilical Cord Stem Cells and Cardiovascular Disease

One of the most frequent causes of cardiovascular disease is inflammation of the left ventricular chamber. Even though there is not necessarily any dysfunction, this condition, called *dilated cardiomyopathy,* often leads to death within five years of diagnosis.

Although higher rates of survival are reported with medication and surgery, the only permanent treatment is a heart transplant, which is risky, rare, and expensive. Recent studies are showing how stem cell therapies are filling the gap and providing a different option for patients.

Research shows that umbilical stem cells "may exert their potential effects not only by the formation of new blood vessels, but also by secreting large amounts of angiogenic, anti-apoptotic, and anti-inflammatory factors."

Research

There are many research articles related to stem cell therapy for cardiovascular disease including the following:

1. Human umbilical cord blood mononuclear cells decrease fibrosis and increase cardiac function in cardiomyopathy

2. Placental mesenchymal and cord blood stem cell therapy for dilated cardiomyopathy
3. Umbilical cord blood-derived mesenchymal stem cells: New therapeutic weapons for idiopathic dilated cardiomyopathy?

You can find the PDFs of the articles on my website www.regenhealthmed.com under patient resources.

COPD

What Is COPD?

Chronic obstructive pulmonary disease, called *COPD*, is the inflammation of the lungs to the point that it restricts airflow. Patients with COPD have difficulty breathing, a constant cough, and a buildup of excessive mucous.

Chronic Obstructive Pulmonary Disease (COPD) defines multiple, different diseases that involve progressive lung damage, including the following:

- **Emphysema:** The air sacs (alveoli) in the lungs become damaged and enlarged, which makes it difficult to push air in and out.
- **Chronic Bronchitis:** Inflammation and mucous buildup in the airway (bronchial tubes) make breathing difficult.
- **Refractory Asthma:** A type of asthma that doesn't respond to medication, where the bronchial tubes swell and tighten.

COPD is most often caused by long-term smoke inhalation. Symptoms do not often appear until considerable damage has been done. Medication and the use of oxygen to assist breathing is common treatment for this disease.

As the disease progresses, the airways become more and more blocked. Patients suffering from COPD face a lack of energy, and often, become bedridden due to weakness and shortness of breath. The inflammation of the lungs is also made worse by pollution, chemicals, and other irritants.

Signs and Symptoms

Not everyone experiences the same symptoms, and COPD displays itself differently, depending on the length and amount of damage that has been done. Of course, a persistent cough is the first, and often, the most obvious, symptom. These are some of the other symptoms:

- Increased dry cough with little relief
- Shortness of breath
- Change in type of breathing, such as wheezing
- Breathlessness or light-headedness
- Excess mucous and phlegm
- Tightness in the throat or chest

Anatomy

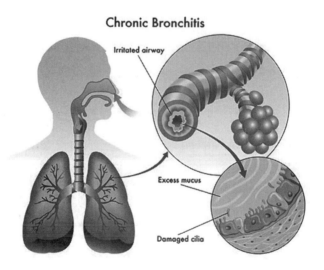

Chronic Bronchitis

Irritated airway

Excess mucus

Damaged cilia

As you can see from the diagram below, the damaged tissue of the lungs creates obstruction and other issues that make proper function problematic.

Risk Factors and Complications

The biggest known risk factor of COPD is smoking. A sizable percentage of smokers end up being diagnosed with one of the types of COPD. Other factors include secondhand smoke, lung irritants like chemical fumes, family history with the AATO gene, and history of respiratory infections as a child.

Previous health conditions or other factors can also complicate or affect COPD in each individual.

Any of the following will change how COPD is managed:

1. High blood pressure
2. Heartburn and digestive issues
3. Heart disease
4. Autoimmune disease
5. Depression or mental health issues

When to Seek Help

People experience coughing and breathing issues for several reasons. From cold, flu, allergy, or irritant, a cough signals the body is fighting some health issue. For the most part, however, coughing is temporary.

If you experience a persistent cough that does not get better, especially up to two weeks later, it is time to seek medical advice. As well, if you have a lingering cough that seems to come and go, it is important to get it looked at.

And, as always, if you experience sudden extreme swelling of the throat or airways, have difficulty breathing or other medical emergency—seek help immediately.

Treatment Options

Care must be taken with people who have some form of COPD that they have their condition monitored by a health-care professional. As the disease progresses, new and different treatment options might need to be considered.

The following is a list of the therapies and treatments that are traditionally used in the medical system to help improve COPD symptoms:

1. **Medications:** Inhalers, steroids, and other anti-inflammatory medications offer relief to many patients.
2. **Lifestyle Changes:** Quitting smoking, changing diet, and physically working on breathing exercises can all improve COPD symptoms.
3. **Oxygen:** As COPD progresses, patients often must carry oxygen to supplement their body's inability to draw in what is required.
4. **Surgery:** In some cases, damaged tissue can be removed from the lungs. For emphysema patients, a surgery to reduce their lung volume often helps. As well, lung transplants are also possible, albeit risky.

Long-Term Outlook

COPD can be experienced in mild to severe forms, depending on a person's symptoms and health history. As well, each disease has its own complications. The long-term outlook for COPD depends on those factors and more.

For treatment and prognosis, COPD is divided into the following stages that are based, among other things, on the percentage of FEV1 (forced expiratory volume), which is the amount of air a person can exhale in one second:

Stage 1: Mild COPD with a near-normal range of FEV1 at around 80 percent

Stage 2: Reduced FEV1 between 50–80 percent

Stage 3: Severe COPD with FEV1 below 50 percent

Stage 4: Extreme COPD with a FEV1 usually below 30 percent, with low blood-oxygen levels.

Why Stem Cell Therapy

The anti-inflammatory properties of stem cell therapy provide an abundance of benefits to patients suffering with COPD. Often, it can be used to address some of the issues that cause or complicate the disease in patients.

As more and more people have discovered, the power of regeneration through stem cell therapy, the opportunities for relief are becoming undeniable.

Stem Cell Therapy for COPD

The medical system currently prescribes medication for COPD that focuses on relieving the symptoms of patients. Up until recently, there were no therapies offered to improve the life of the COPD patient. As stem cell therapy is beginning to be understood, novel regenerative approaches are being investigated.

In the study of the progress of regenerative therapy on COPD, positive results are being discovered. Analyzing the completed clinical trials has shown that there is:

> . . . a new property of stem cells that is potentially capable of curing COPD patients. Small molecules like retinoic acid has

been shown to lead to regeneration and repair of the damaged lung structures in COPD mouse models probably by activation of endogenous lung stem/progenitor cells.

As research continues to progress, and more and more people experience benefits from stem cell therapy for COPD, a deeper understanding of the science of regeneration will be made clear.

Diabetes

Overview of Diabetes

Type 1 diabetes is a degenerative disease where the pancreatic cells are attacked by the immune system. This results in a reduction of insulin production and secretion, and increases the blood sugar level in the body.

Basically, it affects the body's ability to use sugar, since the insulin helps the glucose get into the body's cells. When it is not properly produced, insulin cannot do its job. In this way, diabetes is an autoimmune condition that chronically attacks the pancreas.

Though the cause of this disease is not known, genetic factors affect the likelihood of someone having type 1 diabetes. As well, it is often diagnosed in childhood, which is why it is also known by the name *juvenile diabetes.*

Active research has been ongoing for generations, still the daily injections remain the most common treatment for diabetes. Yet still, there is no long-term or permanent solution, only continued monitoring of the progress.

In **Type 2 diabetes**, your body does not use insulin properly and causes blood glucose (sugar) levels to rise higher than normal. This is also called *hyperglycemia,* or *insulin resistance.* In the beginning stages, your pancreas makes extra insulin to make up for it. But over time, your pancreas isn't able to keep up and can't make enough insulin to keep your blood glucose levels normal.

Type 2 diabetes is the most common form of diabetes. There are about twenty-seven million people in the United States with type 2 diabetes, and another eighty-six million are prediabetic, where their blood glucose is not normal, but not high enough to be diabetic yet.

Type 2 diabetes is treated primarily with lifestyle changes, oral medications (pills), and insulin. If you are an active person and commit to a very healthy-eating lifestyle, often the blood glucose levels can be controlled. You may also need to take prescribed medications or insulin to help you meet your target blood glucose levels. Type 2 usually gets worse over time—even if you don't need medications at first, you may need to take them later on.

When glucose builds up in the blood instead of going into cells, it can starve your cells for energy, and over time, high blood glucose levels may hurt your eyes, kidneys, nerves, or heart.

Some ethnic groups have a higher risk for developing type 2 diabetes than others; it is more commonly diagnosed in African-Americans, Latinos, Native Americans, and Asian-Americans/Pacific Islanders, as well as the aged population. Although not the only contributing factor, being overweight or obese can cause insulin resistance, especially if you carry your extra pounds around the waistline.

Signs and Symptoms

Diabetes is a disease that can have a sudden onset. Often, patients start experiencing some of the following symptoms out of nowhere, when they were previously healthy, with no issues:

- Unquenchable thirst
- Fatigue
- Increased hunger
- Frequent urination
- Unexpected weight loss
- Bed-wetting in children
- Increased irritation and mood swings

Anatomy

Diabetes is a disease that happens when the body is not producing the right levels of insulin. The pancreas, where insulin in the body is made, no longer functions properly.

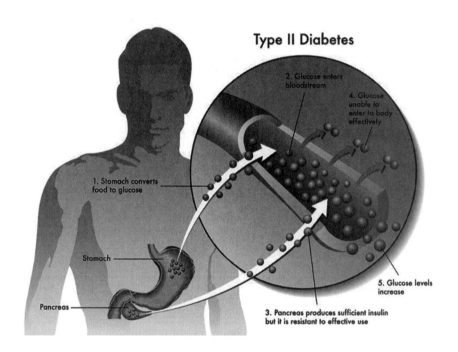

Risk Factors and Complications

Type 1 diabetes affects people across a wide spectrum of ages; however, there are some risk factors that seem to increase the possibility of someone being diagnosed with the disease.

Some of the most identifiable risk factors include the following:

- **Family History:** People with a parent or sibling who has diabetes are more likely to get it themselves.
- **Genetics:** A specific gene has been found to have a correlation to type 1 diabetes.
- **Location:** People who live farther away from the equator are more likely to contract the disease.
- **Age:** Although people of any age can get type 1 diabetes, there is an increased risk during childhood around age eight and then again around age twelve.

When to Seek Help

Low blood sugar, also called *hypoglycemia*, is a serious condition that can lead to hospitalization and death if not treated. Patients with diabetes, as well as their friends and family need to know what symptoms to look for so they can prevent undue harm.

Anyone who is diagnosed with type 1 diabetes and experiences any of the following symptoms should seek help immediately:

- Dizziness and disorientation
- Confusion or behavioral changes
- Seizure
- Loss of consciousness

Treatment Options

To effectively treat diabetes, blood sugar level must be kept as close to normal as possible. This will delay or prevent complications.

Common treatments for type 1 diabetes include the following:

- Insulin injections
- Monitoring diet
- Frequently checking blood sugar level
- Regular exercise

Long-Term Outlook

Diabetes patients begin to have more and more complications as their disease progresses. If they can maintain a balanced blood sugar level, the complications are significantly reduced. Otherwise, as time progresses, the side effects of the disease become severe and even, at times, fatal.

Over the long-term, patients could also experience these conditions:

- High blood pressure and heart disease
- Pain, numbness, and tingling caused by nerve damage
- Kidney damage
- Vision problems
- Poor circulation
- Bacterial and fungal infections, especially on the skin and mouth.

Why Stem Cell Therapy

As patients grow weary of daily insulin injections and continuous degradation of their body's systems, they seek a better way of healing. Science is starting to catch up with the need for alternative therapies for some of the most debilitating conditions.

Stem cell therapy offers regeneration and repair to damaged cells. Studies are beginning to show promise for stem cells to regenerate and replace non-insulin-producing cells, improving the overall health of patients with diabetes.

Karen's Story

"After watching my own mother die early from diabetes-related issues, I saw myself following her path, and it was scary. Losing her was a wake-up call, and I started to reevaluate what I considered part of my life.

"Monitoring my insulin with injections twice a day, feeling worn out, and being unable to lose weight, it was just bad genetics, or so I thought at the time. It seemed I was to follow in my mother's footsteps, and it was a depressing path I was taking.

"Life seemed short, dark, and painful. After a few years of coping with my health issues, my husband left. He wanted someone he could enjoy life with, and I wasn't cutting it. Divorce didn't help my depression, and I had all but given up.

"The thing with diabetes is that no one talks about long-term improvement. The medicine is only to manage symptoms and prolong life, such as it is. Since I saw no reason to look forward, I kept my head down and tried to make it through the day.

"I actually heard about stem cell therapy from the teacher I work with. We share a class and both work half-time. Last year, I just couldn't keep up with a full-time job, so I had to make arrangements for a job share.

"It was a blessing in disguise though, as Becky, the teacher I work with, become a close friend, and I always say she saved my life. One of her relatives had stem cell therapy, and they stopped requiring insulin and got rid of all their symptoms. They said it was a miracle.

"Mostly, I went for it because Becky wouldn't stop bothering me about it. Every day, she asked me if I went for a consultation, so finally I just did it to shock her the next time she asked.

"Turns out, I was the one who was shocked because it changed my whole view in one meeting. The medical professionals actually seemed to care about me, and the information was direct and science-based.

"After the therapy, I didn't get the instant miracle I was half hoping for. But I did begin to see improvement over time. My nerve pain eventually disappeared altogether, and at my last doctor's appointment, my insulin-intake requirements were reduced. I only need one injection per day, which is a big deal for me.

"Overall, I get why people are hesitant. It is not something we hear about that much yet. But once you learn, it makes a lot of sense. Then, you see how it works, and you wonder why you didn't find out about it sooner."

Stem Cell Therapy for Diabetes: From Hype to Hope

The current standard treatment for diabetes is a daily insulin supplement, using an insulin pump or often, multiple injections. Over the years, improvements have been made in glucose monitoring and patient wellness, yet still, the insulin is required. As well, there are complications from the degeneration that are not addressed with the addition of the insulin:

- Retinopathy
- Nephropathy
- Neuropathy

Using past success as a predictor for the future of stem cells on diseases like diabetes, researchers have looked into the promising results of regenerative therapy for patients, stating:

> While the regenerative potential of stem cells can be harnessed to make available a self-replenishing supply of glucose-responsive, insulin-producing cells, their immunomodulatory properties may potentially be used to prevent, arrest, or reverse autoimmunity . . . and prevent recurrence of the disease.

The University of Virginia's study focused on the regenerative properties of stem cells in patients with diabetes. The study looked at therapeutic interventions for diabetes in different, corresponding areas:

- Preservation of cells
- Restoration of glucose-responsiveness
- Replacement and regeneration
- Protection from autoimmune destruction

Research Articles

There are many research articles related to stem cell therapy for diabetes including the following:

1. Status of stem cells in diabetic nephropathy
2. Stem cell therapy to cure type 1 diabetes

You can find the PDFs of the articles on my website www.regenhealthmed.com under patient resources.

Kidney Function

What Is Kidney Function?

Kidney disease happens when damage, degeneration, or other problems are not fairly dealt with. Kidneys have multiple functions that are crucial in the health and well-being of each person, including the following:

- Filters waste and fluid out of the body
- Balances levels of minerals and electrolytes
- Regulates hormones

As the various aspects are moderated, any unnecessary waste is removed through the urine. When the kidneys are not functioning properly, waste builds up, and it can become deadly very quickly.

Common Causes

When the system's functions are not working properly, and the kidneys lose the ability to filter waste from your blood sufficiently, the initial cause might not be obvious. Many different aspects can cause problems to your kidney health and function, such as these:

- Certain chronic diseases like diabetes
- Prolonged dehydration
- Exposure to toxins
- Trauma or injury to the kidneys

Signs and Symptoms

When the kidneys begin to lose functionality, many different symptoms can occur. In some cases, a patient will exhibit no symptoms at all. Other times, it is possible that one or more of these symptoms will be noticed before the kidney function irregularities are detected:

- Fatigue
- Decreased urination
- Fluid retention
- Swollen legs, ankles, and feet
- Shortness of breath
- Nausea and pain
- Pain or pressure in the chest area

Anatomy

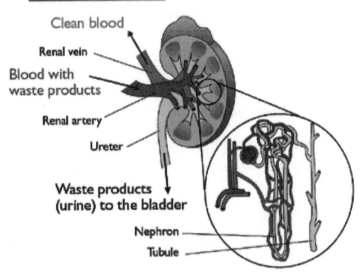

How the kidney works

Diagnosis and Testing

For patients with kidney function problems, doctors can use a variety of different tests to diagnose and discover the problem.

1. **Urinalysis:** Determining the quantity and consistency of the urine provides information about kidney function.

2. **Blood Tests:** Checking for elevated levels of toxins that are usually cleared away during proper kidney function
3. **MRI or Ultrasound:** Giving a visual of the kidneys and checking for any physical damage or other tissue issues

When to Seek Help

Anyone who is worried about proper kidney function should seek medical assistance. Additionally, some of these other issues could be a sign that something is seriously wrong. If any of these issues arise, we recommend you contact your medical team:

- Change in heart rate (very slow or very fast)
- Blood in stool
- Extreme fatigue
- Chest pain

Treatment Options/Surgeries

As kidney function starts to deteriorate, it is monitored quite closely. When the kidney goes into failure, a patient must begin dialysis or have a kidney transplant.

- **Dialysis:** The blood is filtered and purified through a machine that mimics kidney function. Regular dialysis can provide a safe alternative to those whose kidneys no longer function properly.
- **Transplant:** Kidney transplants are required for people who have lost all kidney function. Unfortunately, the wait time and potential complications, including the body rejecting the transplanted organ, make this a dangerous option.

Why Stem Cell Therapy

Stem cell therapy is a restorative healing process. Repair and regeneration of kidney function has been proven by multiple scientific studies. The results are continuing to show a positive correlation between stem cell therapy and an increase in overall quality of life.

Studying Umbilical Cord Stem Cells in Regeneration of Kidney Function

Kidney function is depleted in many patients for reasons such as these:

- Diabetes
- Sepsis
- Degeneration
- Disease
- Injury

Up until recently, the majority of studies using stem cells for renal failure focused on bone marrow stem cells derived from the patient. Umbilical cord blood stem cells have only begun to be used more recently, and based on the science, should be even more effective.

Using groups of rats in a lab, the efficacy of stem cells on kidney function was tested. Compared to control groups, it was noted that there was improvement after four weeks of stem cell treatment, with this conclusion:

> Systematically administered umbilical blood-mobilized human HSCs reduce mortality and promote rapid renal repair and regeneration of the kidney by paracrine mechanisms directed at peritubular capillaries. These findings support human umbilical cord blood, primitive, hematopoietic cells as a promising therapeutic strategy for treatment of acute kidney diseases, and in the prevention of chronic kidney diseases.

Research Articles

There are many research articles related to stem cell therapy for kidney function including the following:

1. Delayed Treatment with Human Umbilical Cord Blood-Derived Stem Cells Attenuates Diabetic Renal Injury
2. Hematopoietic stem cells derived from human umbilical cord ameliorate cisplatin-induced acute renal failure in rats
3. Early, but not late, treatment with human umbilical cord blood-derived mesenchymal stem cells attenuates cisplatin nephrotoxicity through immunomodulation

You can find the PDFs of the articles on my website www.regenhealthmed.com under patient resources.

Spinal Cord Injury

What Is Spinal Cord Injury?

When damage to the spine causes either temporary or permanent alterations in a patient's ability, it is considered a spinal cord injury. Depending on where the injury occurred, the severity and type of symptoms will differ.

Generally, pain and complications can happen at and below the injured area, so legs and feet and nervous system issues are often interrelated. The spinal cord has nerves running through it that are damaged during spinal cord injuries. When this happens, the messages that travel through the nerves are not getting through.

Spinal cord injury is closely tied to chronic pain emanating from the back, shoulders, or hips, depending on the scope of the injury. Numbness, sudden or persistent pain, or loss of sensation are symptoms commonly associated with this condition.

Current medical treatments vary, based on the severity of the injury. Initially, physiotherapy and medication might be enough. Often, cortisone injections come next, followed quickly by surgery, when the injections make the situation worse.

Failed surgery and permanent disability have been the outlook for most patients with spinal cord injuries. That is beginning to change as more and more research is done into regenerative therapies.

Signs and Symptoms

Some of the symptoms of spinal cord injury are specific to the location and type of injury, paralysis, for example, depending on which vertebrae and area of the spine are affected. Other symptoms might come and go, depending on the stress put on the injury.

These are the most common symptoms of spinal cord injury:

- Loss of muscle function
- Reduced flexibility
- Dull ache or pain after standing
- Sharp stabbing pain in a localized area
- Stiffness and discomfort in hips, shoulders, legs, and/or feet
- Change in bowel or bladder function
- Tingling and numbness in hands and/or feet
- Breathing problems

Anatomy

Spinal cord injuries differ, depending where on the spine the injury is located. During injury, damage can be done to the discs, the vertebrae, and the nerves that are connected.

Human Vertebrae Anatomy

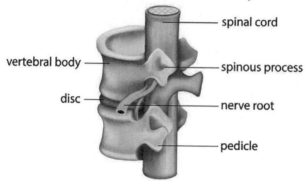

Diagram labels: spinal cord, vertebral body, spinous process, disc, nerve root, pedicle

Diagnosis and Testing

Upon initial consultation, if it is not an emergency, doctors will do a full examination and determine patient history before proceeding with testing. Often people are impatient for a solution, while a doctor may take some time, and potentially, refer the case to a specialized physician for diagnosis.

The physical examination will provide information into how much sensation and movement is lost and to where the patient can proceed. Bloodwork is also completed to get an overall picture of health.

The next step is usually an X-ray to make sure nothing is broken. From there, an MRI or CT scan will show any issue in the soft tissue, ligaments, and discs. This will provide a clearer picture of how the body is reacting to the spinal cord injury.

When to Seek Help

Spinal cord injuries can be serious and life threatening. If you experience any sudden accident or trauma, seek help immediately. Before the injury is assessed, it can be dangerous to even move a person with a spinal cord injury. If there has been an emergency, call 911 and wait for help to arrive.

For ongoing spinal cord issues, if pain gets suddenly worse or there is a serious decline in any of the following, it is important to see a medical professional:

- Movement
- Strength
- Bladder control
- Efficacy of medication

Treatment Options/Surgeries

Spinal cord injury comes in many different forms and affects patients differently. For serious-emergency spinal cord injuries, medical professionals will assess the situation, sometimes on a minute-to-minute basis, just to stabilize the patient.

Other spinal cord injuries are more gradual and might start with a backache and progress from there. When this happens, a doctor starts with a medication to treat the pain, and then moves on to other options depending on the severity of the issue:

- Prescription painkillers
- Nerve blockers
- Steroid injections
- Surgery

Long-Term Outlook

Spinal cord injuries almost always get worse without intervention. Since the spine is holding up the body, there is a lot of stress and strain, and normal activity can be excruciating for people with back problems. Quality of life is greatly reduced over time, as other joints and systems of the body are affected by this type of long-term health issue.

For patients with a spinal cord injury, the usual treatments, and even surgery, do not offer a cure. The structural, muscular, and other health issues continue, even after the original issue has been repaired.

Why Stem Cell Therapy

Spinal cord injury often results in chronic pain. Surgery, injections, and other treatments, even if they fix the mechanical problem, do not address the underlying pain and inflammation. Many treatments and medications worsen the degeneration and problems in the spine.

The benefit of stem cell therapy is that it is not invasive and will not have adverse side effects that could cause more pain or suffering. As well, stem cells have been proven to reduce inflammation and encourage regeneration and repair.

Kevin's Story

"I've worked my whole life as a welder. My grandpa taught me to weld, and he used to weld military airplanes. Me, I stuck to the private sector because it paid more. Working in marine, welding is high demand, and often high risk, but I loved it.

"There'd be me and a couple of guys in the hull of a boat, and it was dark and slippery. The challenging work was the fun stuff, and we would have silly pointless competitions over whose welds were the best.

"We worked together three weeks on, one week off, so we were like a family. Those guys were my best friends, and we hung out after work, talking about the day and making jokes or playing golf.

"One day at work, I fell and hurt my back. It was bad; they had to help me out of the boat. Of course, everyone was pissed because it became a safety issue for them, and there were reports that had to be made. They also got a lot tougher on the safety rules, and everyone blamed me.

"But that wasn't the worst of my problems. I was off work, and the doctor told me to expect not to go back. I had a spinal cord injury, and continuing to weld would aggravate my back and cause stress-related problems.

"At first, I didn't think about not going back; I was in too much pain. But after a while, I missed it. I thought maybe I could just cut my hours back, or the boss could give me something a little easier. The "old guy jobs" as we called them.

"It didn't happen like that though, and all my work friends stopped talking to me. I thought they were just busy, but it wasn't that. I was no longer part of the crew. My boss wouldn't let me come back part-time; in fact, he had a hard time keeping it a secret that he didn't want me back at all.

"So I lost my job and hurt my back again, because I was being stupid. I was helping my brother move, and I wanted to still be the tough guy who didn't need help. But I needed help alright, and the doctors told me I would probably need surgery too.

"It was while I was feeling sorry for myself at my brother's house that his wife asked if I tried stem cell therapy. Of course, I had never heard of it, but I looked into it and decided to just go for it.

"Since then, I have avoided surgery, thankfully. I have also regained strength and reduced my pain. The inflammation and

> *other issues that were worsening my back pain also lessened. Overall, I couldn't believe how smoothly everything went.*
>
> *"From the moment my sister-in-law told me about stem cell therapy, everything fell into place to the path of my healing. I would never in a thousand years have believed I am where I am today, but thanks to this therapy, I am there."*

Stem Cells and Spinal Cord Injury

The *Journal of Hematotherapy & Stem Cell Research* is committed to offering studies on the science and research of stem cell therapy. Spinal cord injury often has multiple, interrelated issues from the nervous system to the muscular system and beyond.

A recent study looked at the ability of stem cells to move to areas in the body and adapt as needed:

> The results suggest that cord blood stem cells are beneficial in reversing the behavioral effects of spinal cord injury, even when infused five days after injury. Human cord blood-derived cells were observed in injured areas, but not in noninjured areas, of rat spinal cords, and were never seen in corresponding areas of spinal cord of noninjured animals. The results are consistent with the hypothesis that cord blood-derived stem cells migrate to and participate in the healing of neurological defects caused by traumatic assault.

The study showed significant improvement in a variety of areas including the following:

- Spinal cord compression
- Inflammation
- Degeneration
- Movement
- Nervous system function

The significance of learning about the migratory aspects of stem cells is just beginning. For conditions with multiple issues, like spinal cord injury, the ability for stem cells to move to the location where they are needed is one that will require more study and holds great promise.

Research Articles

There are many research articles related to stem cell therapy for spinal cord injury including the following:

1. Cellular supplementation technologies for painful spine disorders
2. A case study of a spinal cord-injured patient
3. Human umbilical cord blood stem cells infusion in spinal cord injury

You can find the PDFs of the articles on my website www.regenhealthmed.com under patient resources.

Skin Trauma/Wound Healing

What Is Skin Trauma?

Skin trauma happens regularly as part of everyday life. Our skin is our body's largest organ, and it is prone to scratches, nicks, cuts, and bites from various things in our environment. For the most part, the skin is designed to heal itself efficiently with no long-term damage.

As we all know, aging slows down the process, so wounds on the skin take longer to heal. Infection or repeated irritation can make the problem worse until it becomes a persistent sore.

The natural process that increases skin trauma and prolongs wound-healing time can be mitigated, so it seems, through stem cell therapy.

Common Causes

Skin trauma and wounds happen, that is a given. When a wound does not heal, after an extended period of time, there could be something else going on.

These are some of the most common underlying causes that prevent wound healing:

- Infection
- Diabetes
- Autoimmune condition
- Repetitive irritation
- Inadequate nutrition
- Edema (fluid accumulation)
- Ulcers (open sores that destroy surface tissue)
- Burns

Signs and Symptoms

Typically, skin trauma heals naturally on its own. Our body has the ability to regenerate skin cells and heal wounds. To determine whether your wound or skin injury is not healing properly, assess your condition based on the following symptoms:

1. **Duration:** No improvement in condition after four weeks
2. **Dry Skin or Other Skin Lesions:** Shows overall difficulty in healing
3. **Discharge:** Constant fluid coming from the wound that does not stop

Anatomy

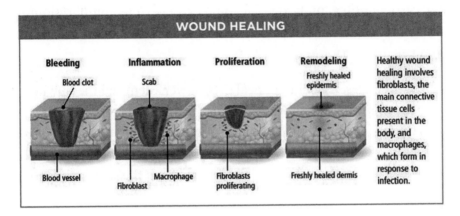

WOUND HEALING

Bleeding	Inflammation	Proliferation	Remodeling	Healthy wound healing involves fibroblasts, the main connective tissue cells present in the body, and macrophages, which form in response to infection.
Blood clot	Scab		Freshly healed epidermis	
Blood vessel	Fibroblast Macrophage	Fibroblasts proliferating	Freshly healed dermis	

Diagnosis and Treatment

When a wound does not heal, a doctor will look for the underlying reasons why.

There are a few different treatment options available for people who have a problem with open wounds:

1. **Topical Ointments:** Medication is often prescribed to prevent infection and encourage healing.
2. **Oxygen Therapy:** Increased oxygen increases rate of collagen and healing properties.
3. **Ultrasound Treatment:** This option uses vibration to stimulate the cells around the wound. It also improves circulation.
4. **Magnetic Therapy:** This option is said to boost circulation and relieve pain while encouraging regrowth of skin cells.

When to Seek Help

If you have a deep wound or an injury where there is something embedded in the skin, it is essential to seek help to prevent infection. As well, if there is redness that spreads, swelling, or tenderness, that could be a sign that an infection is spreading.

It is also important to seek medical attention, if you have a blood disease or another condition that could cause serious complications.

Why Stem Cell Therapy

As our skin ages, its ability to heal gets slower. Stem cell therapy helps the body rejuvenate and leads to swifter healing and recovery. The way stem cells regenerate reduces inflammation and repairs damaged tissue, making it an ideal choice to improve skin trauma. Often patients see wounds healing, when they initially had received the stem cell therapy for another condition.

Stem Cell Therapy in Wound Healing

The study of tissue damage and regeneration is making remarkable progress as research is being done on the effective therapies for treatment.

Regeneration after injury or damage to skin requires multiple changes in cellular behavior including the following:

- Initiating wound healing
- Mitigating cell death
- Differentiation of cells
- Integration of regenerated tissue

Researchers studying the process are seeing:

Wound-healing therapies continue to rapidly evolve, with advances in basic science and engineering research heralding the development of new therapies, as well as ways to modify existing treatments. Stem cell-based therapy is one of the most promising therapeutic concepts for wound healing.

This and other ongoing studies show the benefit of stem cell therapy in areas that require multiple process and growth factors involved in healing. As research continues, the use of stem cell therapy in skin trauma and wound healing will continue to become more and more effective.

Research

There are many research articles related to stem cell therapy for skin trauma and wound healing, including the following:

1. Role of cord blood mesenchymal stem cells in recent deep burn
2. The use of stem cells in burn wound healing
3. Clinical trial of human umbilical cord blood-derived stem cells for the treatment of moderate-to-severe atopic dermatitis:

You can find the PDFs of the articles on my website www.regenhealthmed.com under patient resources.

Stroke/Traumatic Brain Injury

What Is a Stroke or Brain Injury?

A stroke is a brain injury that happens when a clot creates a blockage in the blood supply to the brain. The longer it lasts, the more cells die off. When oxygen supply is cut off to the brain, it only takes a few minutes for cells to die off and a loss of function to occur. Where and how this shows itself as symptoms, depends on where the blood clot is located.

These are the most common symptoms of stroke:

- Difficulty speaking
- Trouble hearing or understanding
- Sudden weakness
- Paralysis (inability to move)
- Numbness or drooping of the face, arms, or legs

Strokes and other traumatic brain injuries are medical emergencies and need to be treated as such. Although stroke is the leading cause of death in the United States, new therapies are being pursued that reduce damage and are seeing patients regain some of their health freedoms, using stem cell therapy after recovery.

Common Causes

There are multiple risk factors that increase the chance of having a stroke. Good health and lifestyle choices are a large part of reducing that risk.

These are some of the common causes of stroke:

- Brain injury
- Smoking
- Tumor
- High blood pressure
- Lack of exercise
- Diabetes
- Poor blood circulation
- Increased stress
- Heart disease

Anatomy

Types of Stroke

Ischemic stroke

Blocked blood vessel

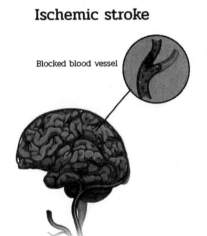

Hemorrhagic stroke

Ruptured blood vessel

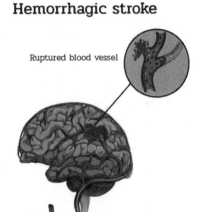

Diagnosis and Testing

For each individual, it will depend not only on the type of stroke sustained, but when it is discovered and how serious it is. Often, a stroke is caught while it is happening, and emergency personnel address the situation as they see it.

Usually, it is after the stroke that testing is done to decipher what symptoms and side effects have occurred. At this time, doctors will also look at underlying causes of the stroke to prevent it from happening again.

Blood tests to check specific issues are completed, along with a physical exam. After that, a CT scan or MRI is often completed to determine the extent of the damage to brain tissue.

When to Seek Help

Strokes are deadly serious, life-threatening health concerns. These are the warning signs of stroke that cannot be ignored:

- Numbness or weakness on one side of the body (face, arm, leg)
- Dizziness, loss of balance
- Sudden severe headache
- Trouble seeing
- Difficulty speaking or understanding speech

If you experience any of these early symptoms, seek help immediately.

Treatment Options/Surgeries

Most of the time, treatment is reactionary in an emergency situation. Anticlotting medication can be given, often through IV, to reduce the severity of the stroke. Other times, medicine is injected straight into the brain. For strokes that involve bleeding in the brain, steps are taken to relieve pressure and stop the bleeding.

After a stroke occurs, the focus is on rehabilitation and repair. Surgery is sometimes an option to repair blood vessels. Physical therapy and rehabilitation are the primary goals, so that patients can regain as much control over their bodies as possible.

Long-Term Outlook

Depending on the severity of the stroke, people can experience long-term recovery and management of their symptoms. By following specific treatments and lifestyle options, the outlook for patients who have experienced a stroke is extremely beneficial.

Why Stem Cell Therapy

A stroke is, in effect, brain damage. As with the other conditions we discussed in this book, stem cell therapy provides regeneration to damaged muscle and tissue. The anti-inflammatory properties and the healing and repairing that stem cells naturally accomplish can do a lot to improve some of the difficult health issues facing patients who have suffered from a stroke.

Ray - Suffering with Debilitating Headaches After Stroke

When I came to get a stem cell injection for knee pain, I was 64 years old and I had been suffering with for more than 40 years. Now my knee feels incredible, but the side benefit I had not even thought to expect was a headache I had daily since I had a stroke a few years back.

After 48 hours of the stem cell injection my headache subsided. I have been headache free except for a two-hour period that was manageable and subsided on its own.

That might not seem like a big deal to everyone but for me it has been unbelievable mentally and physically. Beforehand, I had constant pain in my head all day, every day. It is amazing what happened, especially because no one expected it. And the improvement has been really life changing. My neurologist even finally gave credit when he reduced the amount of pills I was taking.

Before the stem cell therapy, I would get headaches in three different areas.

1. It felt like a nail to my left temple.
2. A stabbing pain above my right eye that rendered me immobile.
3. There was an almost constant pain that felt like I was being sliced along my head.

No pills worked on the first two types of headaches and they stopped me in my tracks. I could not be in the room with others and I had to sit or lie down in darkness until they subsided.

I came to Dr. Banerjee to fix my knee and had no idea my headaches would be relieved. Now if I get a small headache, it is every 10-20 days and it is minimal. My knee strength is so much better and I never wake up with knee pain. I tend to overdo it once in a while in the yard but then I wake up I feel better, I can rest and recover more quickly.

Over the past six weeks since I had the therapy, I have begun to do the things I could not previously do. Over the last few decades I have had my knee scoped and treated and finally 40 years after the injury I am getting pain free movement.

Another little added benefit was something that I had just been living with, for years. I suffered from a hand injury about 15 or so years ago. I wasn't able to grip a golf club and my hand was a bit swollen and it was just something I lived with even though it acted up and made certain tasks more difficult.

Then a week or so after the stem cell treatment, I was surprised to open a jar without pain. Then it dawned on me that the pain was quite a bit reduced and my hand was no longer swollen. I pointed it out to my wife and she couldn't believe it. She said it was like the stem cell therapy from the inside out and I my body seemed to be regenerating.

So, after only one knee injection I have seen benefits in three different areas. It has far surpassed my expectations and now I have my father ready to get stem cell therapy.

Timing of Stem Cell Therapy after Stroke

Every three minutes, someone dies from a stroke according to the American Stroke Association. According to a study by the University of South Florida, stem cell therapy can improve a stroke patient's symptoms significantly, depending on when it is given.

According to this research, if the therapy was given in response to inflammation caused by stroke, the timing made all the difference. If it occurred earlier or later than this window, then no benefit accrued, and in some cases, recovery was impeded: *"The timing of treatment is more important than the dose of cells because the effective dose at forty-eight hours is an order of magnitude smaller than the optimal dose at earlier time points."*

The results indicate that stem cell therapy given too soon after a stroke, inhibits or confuses the body's natural defenses and potentially causes more damage. As well, when therapy is given too many days after a stroke, the resulting benefits will be minimal. As research continues to pinpoint the most effective therapies, improvements in stroke recovery and other conditions will become more successful.

Research

There are many research articles related to stem cell therapy for stroke and traumatic brain injuries including the following:

1. Intra-arterial transplantation of human umbilical cord blood mononuclear cells in hyperacute stroke improves vascular function
2. Intravenous Administration of Human Umbilical Cord Blood Reduces Behavioral Deficits After Stroke in Rats
3. Timing of Cord Blood Treatment After Experimental Stroke Determines Therapeutic Efficacy

You can find the PDFs of the articles on my website www.regenhealthmed.com under patient resources.

CHAPTER 6

Answering Your Questions about Stem Cell Therapy

Putting the Patient First

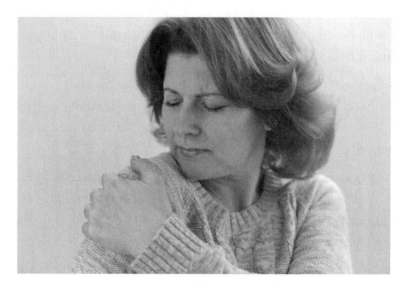

The whole reason this book was written is the sad fact that putting the patient first is not the common process in mainstream health care, for the most part. The system is prioritized first, and the patient must fit in. In this way, it is much harder to find relevant information about your health and how the body works toward healing.

When patients are experiencing pain and suffering from their condition, they are mostly concerned with questions that will expedite their healing process. By addressing concerns that touch on the top inquiries we receive, people are better able to make decisions for their own health.

Most often, questions and concerns usually deal with something related to one of the following:

- Finances
- Speed of healing
- Risks or safety

I want to make sure you have everything clear from the outset. It is the only way to provide professional and consistent health care, and there is no better time than now to stand up for your own body's needs and find out as much information as you can.

By getting clear and concise answers to the questions that most people have, you can get to the point of understanding, so you can move forward to a better life for yourself. One of the greatest attributes of stem cell therapy is the transparency.

Every single *who, what, when, where,* and *why* answer is laid out in a regulated process designed to meet the needs of the patient. We want to put the answers in terms you understand, so you can know how it will look for your specific situation.

For some people, the answers might be different, based on their medical condition and overall health. That is why we offer a consultation, because it is much more prudent to discuss the personal aspects of each individual's situation, one-on-one.

Our answers to the most common, frequently asked questions, which we address in this chapter, offer insight into the safety and efficacy of stem cell therapy, including the perspectives of the patients who have been there. Hearing stories and seeing what and how things are done is the first step in finding out if stem cell therapy is right for you.

Carl's Story—Looking for Answers

"My message is clear, but it took me long enough to figure it out—don't knock it until you try it. When I first heard about stem cell therapy, I wanted to know as much about it as possible, but I found conflicting information. What exactly was stem cell therapy, and why were people freaking out about it?

"There were some aspects of the controversy that seemed to ignore basic science, and I knew there had to be more to the story. I am usually quite a skeptic.

"My bad knee gave me the gift of a lot of time to look into things. I had an injury from years ago, and every now and then, it would get worse, and worse. As time went on, I tried every different physical therapy and medication that was offered to me, but none of it worked, except the pain pills.

"And the pain pills worked too well. I could see myself using them when I didn't need to, just to get the feel-good response. Fortunately, my doctor called me on it when I wanted him to up my dose. He showed me enough to know I had to curb my usage of these pills before they became an addiction.

"Everyone does things their own way, and I went cold turkey. Knowing myself, I had to do it just like when I stopped smoking. Decide enough is enough and just never do it again. It wasn't easy, but I kept to myself and spent a lot of time looking up stories of other people like me, to inspire me to keep going.

"YouTube is great for that because everyone has a chance to tell their story. And I could sit there and search different options, while I tried to keep my mind off my knee and those pills.

"It was during this time that I kept hearing about stem cells in conversation with people about natural health care or alternative options that worked for them. So I tried to find out more in order to make the connection as to why some people were saying it was so good, while others said it was so bad.

"Then, when I heard Mel Gibson talking about and supporting stem cell therapy, I started to look into it a little more deeply. I think it was because he shared his message about his dad and then other people, himself included, had also experienced benefits from stem cell therapy and how they felt was much better.

"I mean, he is not the kind of guy that needs to endorse something, so it's like there is some credibility there. At the same time, I am not the kind of guy that jumps into something just because a celebrity told me to.

"When I went looking for answers, they were right there. It is kind of sad that I had been used to not getting answers. Doctors I went to, and even random people who heard about my knee problem, had advice, but when you ask them why, they didn't know. The medical system dictates answers, it doesn't discuss them.

"So when my questions were answered, with science to back them up, I couldn't believe it. The people I spoke with were professional and clearly expressed the process and procedure, the follow up, and anything else I could think to ask.

"Afterward, they followed up with me regularly and monitored my progress. It helped me document how much improvement I had made.

"My knee had dictated my life previously and really limited where I could go. My daughter and her husband had this new, gorgeous,

beachfront property, and I couldn't go see them because of the number of stairs I had to climb to get there.

"In fact, I was becoming the family joke—the crazy, old, conspiracy guy, sitting in front of his computer, watching YouTube. I may have added to that with my insistence that the medical system was corrupt.

"The whole ordeal was becoming quite horrible, starting with my experience with the painkillers. Now, with no medication, I was apt to be grouchy and uncomfortable all the time. Knowing how quickly I snapped, I just pushed everyone away to avoid it.

"It was devastating, and I hated how, at the same time, it made me rely on other people for everything. When your knee doesn't hurt, you don't realize how much it affects everything you do. For me, it was one little twist, and my knee was never the same again. The pain is not just in the knee either; it shoots up and down the body and causes other issues that start to pile up.

"My body wasn't my own anymore, and I was angry that I had become an old man so soon. My wife stopped coming to the doctor's appointments with me, because I was always grouchy for days afterward because nothing was helping.

"I did all the research I could about stem cell therapy, so when anyone called me nuts, I had something to prove otherwise. It's funny though, because no one laughed.

"I will never forget the day I climbed up to see my daughter's new house and join in a big family barbeque. The sight is one I will never forget, and the ocean never looked so good. Everyone else wanted to know what my secret was, and I was just sitting there, thankful to be with my family.

> "It shouldn't be a secret; stem cell therapy is actually safe, effective, and amazing. At least, it was for me. The trouble is with the reporting of what stem cell therapy is all about; there is some false news or incomplete information being shared."

Your Frequently Asked Questions

It is always our intention to ensure transparency and knowledge from the get-go with all patients. In writing this book, I want to make sure all of your questions are answered, and we do not avoid anything, even the tough questions.

You can also follow the resources provided throughout the book, as the science and regulatory practices are well documented elsewhere. Of course, it is always recommended to seek out the opinion of the professionals and people you trust.

They will likely have some of the same questions you do and many of the answers are contained in this book. Also, if you want more information on one or more of these questions contact us at www.RegenHealthMed.com.

We appreciate your feedback and questions at any time, as we seek to provide this information to patients looking for different healing solutions.

What Are Stem Cells?

Answer: All parts of our bodies are made up of cells that work together to keep us alive.

Scientists discovered that certain cells, like stem cells, are the building blocks of all other cells and provide regeneration.

Stem cells are called *undifferentiated* because they have not yet determined a function. These are unique cells that initiate life by dividing into cells that become specialized.

Picture it like a blank canvas—when a stem cell divides, the new cells are able to adapt to the function required of them. In this way, a body grows cells for the different systems required to sustain life. As the stem cells divide, they form new stem cells, as well as cells with a very specific function.

Stem cells develop to form different cells in the body such as the following:

- Liver
- Brain
- Tissue
- Blood
- Lungs
- Nerves
- Heart
- Bone
- Liver
- Muscle

The significance of this is in seeing the results of additional stem cells on a patient. When one or more parts of a person's body are struggling, the stem cells can adapt to exactly what is needed to improve the situation.

Remarkable results are being seen in a vast assortment of conditions and diseases. Patients from around the world are describing how stem cell therapy has helped them live a longer, healthier, pain-free life.

At the same time, rapid research and new innovations into stem cell technology are being studied worldwide. Although stem cell therapy is still somewhat new, the process is proven, tested, and safe. In reality, it has been around for over three decades.

Stem Cell Therapy for Athletes

Before stem cell therapy became readily available, it was highly sought out, but rarely spoken about. For more than ten years, while most people didn't even have it on their radar, thousands of athletes and movie stars have been using stem cell therapy. In fact, Jack Nicklaus has been using stem cell therapies for years.

Throughout his career, Jack Nicklaus suffered severe back pain. He underwent many different treatments from steroid injections to back surgery, and yet nothing helped. His condition slowly worsened. Although he did not see immediate results, he noticed, after receiving the procedure, his pain slowly subsided. He has gone back for more stem cell therapy and said, "I'm not a doctor, but I think that stem cell [therapy] is going to change . . . the direction of orthopedics, totally."

Other athletes, looking for more swift and thorough healing for ongoing injuries, have been quietly seeking out stem cell therapy for improvement in sports-related injuries. The practice is becoming so common in some sports that teams harvest and store stem cells from their players for use in injuries throughout the season.

These are other well-known athletes who have reportedly received stem cell therapy:

- Tennis star Rafael Nadal
- Chiefs running back Jamaal Charles
- Braves pitcher Bartolo Colon
- Spurs forward Pau Gasol
- Redskins tight end Jordan Reed
- Retired quarterback Peyton Manning

Hockey legend, Gordie Howe, underwent stem cell therapy after a stroke left him unable to walk or speak. He required continuous care and spent much of his time in bed, unresponsive. After stem cell therapy, he regained his ability to speak and was able to walk again. Previously, his family was planning his funeral, as he was in such quick decline. His remarkable recovery made headlines, as he was able to, once again, attend and take part in public events.

These are just a few of the many well-known athletes and celebrities seeking out regenerative medicine and seeing benefits from a wide variety of health conditions, through the healing properties of stem cell therapy. As the procedure becomes more and more accepted, we will likely hear of others who use the same approach to health care.

When Jack Nicklaus was asked why he did not talk about his stem cell therapy, he replied that it was because no one asked. This really sheds light on the procedure overall, as for so long, it was not well understood or talked about. Fortunately, that is beginning to change.

What Is the Difference between Autologous Stem Cells and Allogeneic Stem Cells?

Answer: These two stem cell types are very different.

1. Autologous stem cells come from the patient that is going to receive them.
2. Allogeneic stem cells come from a donor (i.e. human umbilical cord tissue stem cells).

What Are Embryonic Stem Cells?

Answer: When a patient is choosing stem cell therapy, the stem cells themselves can come from one of a number of different sources. It is important to determine from where the stem cells are sourced and what that means. There are special issues to consider for each source.

Stem cell therapy that uses embryonic stem cells sources the cells from human embryos. An embryo is a human fertilized egg from the initial cell division until the end of the eighth week of gestation. After that, the embryo is considered a fetus.

When embryonic stem cells are taken, the embryo is destroyed. The majority of these stem cells come from IVF (in vitro fertilization) facilities and are leftover embryos that were initially created for reproductive purposes.

Since the stem cells have an unlimited ability for regeneration, they have been used for tissue replacement, autoimmune diseases, and other conditions. At that stage of development, the cells can easily differentiate for use in many different areas.

The debate most people raise is as to when life is considered to exist. If the embryo becomes a fetus, what exactly is being destroyed? All of these are valid concerns that are beyond the scope of this book.

In our practice, **we DO NOT use embryonic stem cells.** The ethical issues alone are not worth pursuing this source of stem cells. As well, the stem cells from umbilical cord blood have the same properties without the potential loss of life.

As I have previously mentioned, our clinic uses the stem cells from umbilical cord blood, which are obtained from a highly reputable company. Our reason for choosing umbilical cord blood is based on the scientific studies, and the experience and feedback of clients.

Having a safe and consistent supply of abundant stem cells provides us with the ability to offer dependable treatment, tailored to the needs of the patient. It is imperative to our health-care services that we offer only safe and ethical procedures.

The stem cells we use are chosen to prevent some of the issues that occur with other stem cell therapies like the following:

- Potential for allergic reaction
- Low quantity of stem cells based on age or illness
- Complications from a live donor
- Reduced efficiency of older stem cells over time
- Potential ethical issues, depending on where stem cells are sourced
- Possible contamination or unhealthy stem cells

"Umbilical cord blood is blood that remains in the placenta and in the attached umbilical cord after childbirth. Cord blood is collected because it contains stem cells, which can be used to treat hematopoietic and genetic disorders."

CORD BLOOD—WIKIPEDIA

	Umbilical Cord Blood HSCs	Bone Narrow HSCs	Under Mobilized peripheral blood HSCs
Ease of collection	No safety risk for mother or child	Donor needs to be anesthetized proceedure in the OP, takes several hours	Requires mobilization causing some discomfort to the donor
Time to engraft	Median time of 3 weeks	Median time of 16-18 days	Median time of 13-15 days
Viral Infections	Rare	Common	Common
Graft vs host diseases (GvHD)	Uncommon and Less severe even if there is GvHD	Common in mismatched grafts	More risk of chronic GvHD than with bone marrow
HLA matching	HLA mismatch well tolerated	Requires a perfect HLA-match	Requires a perfect HLA-match
Repeat Transplant	Not Possible	Possible	Possible
HSC numbers	Low, hence poor engraftment	High, hence poor engraftment	High, hence poor engraftment

What Are the Steps to Treatment?

Answer: The first step toward stem cell therapy is education. As a patient, you need to know what stem cell therapy is and how it will work for you and your healing process. As a doctor, I want you to know what I do, so you can proceed with positivity.

After the initial consultation, there are certain tests that need to be done. We look at your condition from a holistic perspective and offer a stem cell therapy procedure, tailored to fit your exact needs. Once we know what that means for you, all the arrangements can be made.

This is when the stem cell therapy is scheduled. It is a noninvasive procedure and should take no more than fifteen minutes from start to finish. You should be able to return to light, daily activity and some patients see an improvement immediately.

Around six weeks afterward, you will be seen for a follow-up appointment to gauge progress. By this time, most patients already have seen significant improvements. Often, patients will decide to have stem cell therapy in another area because they have seen such great results.

In any case, you will have professional guidance from before you decide to try stem cell therapy until long after the procedure takes place.

What Does the Treatment Cost?

Answer: The cost of stem cell therapy depends on your condition and the treatment you will need. Each dose differs for each patient.

Call our office to schedule an evaluation. We will inform you of our next live seminar. We will also send you a stem cell seminar video that will answer 99% of the questions you may have.

That being said, our team will go through the exact costs at the time of the initial consultation. All scenarios will be discussed and all questions will be answered to ensure you are completely comfortable with all aspects of the treatment.

When compared to surgery or long-term medication and health-care treatments, the cost is very reasonable. When you consider how important your quality of life really is and the many more activities you will be able to do as a result of having no pain, the costs are insignificant.

How Many Treatments Will I Need?

Answer: The number of treatments needed is specific to an individual. Many people find one treatment is all that is necessary, if their degenerative condition is not overly advanced. At the same time, this is dependent on the individual.

Since stem cell therapy treats such a wide variety of conditions, diseases, and areas of the body, it depends on personal variables. Often, patients who see benefits from the first round of stem cell therapy choose to have more in order to see that improvement increase.

Other times, patients have one procedure, and their life improves substantially, so that they have other areas of their health they also want to improve. Once again, it is a very personal choice.

Does Insurance Cover This?

Answer: Stem cell therapy is not covered by insurance, because insurance does not normally cover natural health treatments. It is considered very affordable in comparison to treatments covered by health insurance.

For most patients, their health has no price, and they are surprised that the true cost of stem cell therapy is much lower than they anticipated. We now offer patient financing with zero money down, upon credit qualification, to be paid back over twenty-four months with no interest. It is a no-brainer to get the stem cell therapy done, if finances are a concern.

Everything is covered in the seminar, and all your questions are answered concerning financing. You can also watch the webinar on my website: www.RegenHealthMed.com for more information.

What Conditions Can Stem Cell Therapy Be Used For?

Answer: Stem cells are a regenerative medicine and work in areas of the body that require healing. That is a broad statement, but it is the truth. The conditions stem cells can be used for are as varied as each patient that comes in seeking answers.

To get a little more specific, stem cell therapy is particularly effective in patients who are experiencing inflammation or degeneration.

These are some of the conditions about which we most often hear the most enthusiastic feedback from patients who see improvements:

- Knee pain
- Autoimmune issues
- Diabetes
- Arthritis
- Skin and tissue damage
- Cardiovascular issues
- Shoulder pain
- Spinal cord injury
- Organ function
- Hip problems

How Long Will It Take to Recover?

Answer: There is no significant recovery time required for stem cell therapy. The procedure is noninvasive and completed in the clinic; most patients return to a lighter version of their regular duties the next day.

In some cases, patients feel tenderness in the area of the procedure. This is usually minimal and does not last long. Muscle spasm or a light ache may be present for a few days and can be alleviated with ice.

Since stem cells have an anti-inflammatory aspect to them, people often feel a reduction in pain immediately. In this way, many patients feel better immediately after stem cell therapy. It is important to take it easy, especially if you see an immediate improvement. Use caution with any activity for the first few weeks, just to give the stem cells a chance to do their job without added stress.

How Long Does It Take to See Results?

Answer: Results are varied from individual to individual. Many patients report improvement in the first week or two. Others report a noticeable difference in only a few days. Since stem cells replicate repeatedly, results can continue to increase for seven months to a year, because the body is regenerating that whole time.

There are some people who see only a small improvement after their first stem cell therapy and then see greater results after the next procedure, all depending on your age, your weight, and how much inflammation and damage you have in your body. Each condition or disease requires different follow-up and time, and the severity of each person's health plays a part in it as well. This will be discussed thoroughly during your consultation.

What Symptoms Improve after Stem Cell Therapy?

Answer: Each condition, each patient, and each procedure are a little bit different, and no results are guaranteed. In fact, it is expected that each person will react differently, based on the individual's symptoms, health history, and several other factors.

Out of all the case studies and client stories from patients who have seen benefits from stem cell therapy, these are the most common improvements noted:

- Decreased pain
- Increased stamina and mobility
- Mentality clarity and energy
- Feeling of rejuvenation

Are There Any Dietary Requirements before, during, and after Stem Cell Therapy?

Answer: There are no special rules for what you can and cannot eat or drink at any time during stem cell therapy. Since it is a noninvasive, in-office procedure, no fasting is required. Of course, each patient has different conditions being treated, and it is best to consult with your doctor for any further direction.

As well, there are some suggestions that will be made as part of your healing plan that may involve dietary restrictions. These work in conjunction with the stem cell therapy to put the patient on track to a whole-health overhaul. In this case, as well, each individual patient will consult with the health-care team to ensure the correct information is received.

If you are looking for specifics on dietary changes and lifestyle management after stem cells, look into our stem cell enhancement program outlined in chapter 8.

How Long Will the Results Last?

Answer: Once again, there is not one set answer for what results will be seen and how long they will last. People usually fall into one of three categories when it comes to determining how long the results last:

1. **Immediate results seen by patients**
   - A percentage of people feel better in the first few days after receiving stem cell therapy.
   - Usually the results also increase over time for these patients, so the initial changes get stronger over time.

2. **Results start to show three weeks after therapy**
   - It is very common for patients to start to see improvement around three weeks after therapy as it takes time for the stem cells to do their work.
   - This also depends on the condition and health of the patient, everyone is different.
3. **Gradual change beyond six weeks**
   - Other times it takes much longer for a patient to experience improvement after stem cell therapy.
   - This includes people who have very gradual results as well as those who might not notice a substantial change.
   - For some, the positive changes in their body are not immediately noticed.

It is important to note that there are no typical results, and every patient is assessed on an individual basis.

Is Stem Cell Therapy Approved?

Answer: Since stem cell therapy is not a medication, it cannot be approved by the U.S. Food and Drug Administration (FDA). Yet the stem cells that are used are rigorously tested and processed, based on FDA regulations.

There are also other agencies such as the American Association of Blood Banks, the National Institute of Health, and the World Health Organization that monitor and oversee the process and procedures involved in stem cell therapy.

Is Stem Cell Therapy Safe?

Answer: Stem cell therapy is safe. Every organ and cell in your body has stem cells in it, so it is a natural aspect of the healing process. The stem cells we use are safely sourced from human umbilical cord blood. They are transported and kept under rigidly regulated processes to ensure safety and efficacy throughout.

The medical process of using stem cells has been happening for a significant number of years. When blood transfusions begin in early World War I, those were a form of stem cell therapy. Since then, the research and independent studies have verified the safety of stem cell therapy.

Compare Stem Cells to Surgery

But there are risks to actually having surgery. It is not just the surgery price itself—it is what you can lose from the surgery as well.

The mother of one of my good friends had knee arthroscopic surgery on Christmas eve. On Christmas day, she died from a blood clot. Another friend had two knee replacements, and then, ended up with kidney failure, having to go on dialysis.

So you don't know what can happen during surgery

In my opinion stem cell therapy is a much better option than surgery.

What Are the Risks?

Answer: Stem cell therapy is safe and highly regulated. Tens of thousands of umbilical cord stem cell therapies have been undertaken in clinics across the United States with no ill effects.

A few patients report feeling mild symptoms for a day or two after the therapy such as these:

- Nausea
- Numbness

- Minor fever
- Headache
- Fatigue
- Infection

If any of these do happen, they are likely to be quite small, and less problematic. Major or permanent risks just do not occur with our stem cells, as we keep everything as simple as possible throughout the entire process.

In reality, none of my patients have experienced these complaints, and most times, they get off the table, drive back home, and experience no ill side effects.

Where Are the Umbilical Cord Cells Obtained From?

And other related questions: Is it an accredited commercial source of banked cord blood? What screening procedures are done for donors?

Answer: The stem cells that we use come from human umbilical cord cells. When women consent to donate umbilical cord blood, they are rigorously tested to ensure they are healthy. Our lab is a FDA- and CA-registered tissue bank. The cells are tested for infectious diseases (HIV, Lyme, Chagas, Hep B and C, CMV, syphilis, HTLV, West Nile). The donors are tested in a CLIA-licensed lab (Clinical Laboratory Improvement Amendments), using antibody tests and PCR-based tests (polymerase chain reaction). Microbial testing is performed, also. They exceed the current guidelines.

Once the stem cells have been obtained, they are fully tested. No chemicals are added. The pure stem cells are washed, then rinsed, and frozen.

Umbilical cord tissue from healthy birthed babies and healthy mothers, which is the safest and least invasive method of extraction available.

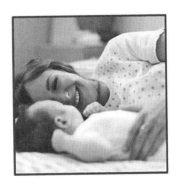

What Screening Procedures Are Used to Determine Safety of Stem Cells?

And other related questions: Does screening include, for example, HIV, HPV, HCV, oncogenic mutations, and other genetic mutations that may be linked to the propensity to develop autoimmune disease? Is this information provided to the patient for the batch of cells that will be injected?

Answer: Predictive Biotech ensures accuracy and testing, and that is where we obtain our stem cells. They have a flow cytometry machine that counts the viable cells, and we also have third-party lab testing that verifies stem cell count. As well, they maintain specific documentation on all of the stem cell products. Each tissue is recorded and separated into controlled lots and quarantined and stored in a cryotank at -196 degrees.

The donating mother has extensive behavioral and health screenings (and is a volunteer donor). Cells are NOT pooled between different donors. Every vial of cells has a donor identification number and bar code, so every vial can be traced from donor to recipient. Every vial is quarantined at the lab until we know that the disease and microbial testing has been successfully completed. We have additional quality-control testing for cell viability and cell size. Our lab is an FDA- and CA-registered tissue bank.

What Viral Screening Is Employed to Screen for Latent Viruses?

And other related questions: Regarding viruses integrated into the DNA, for example: Were the stem cells derived from a mother who was a drug addict and what was her health status?

Answer: Stem cells inherently do not have any mechanisms to directly alter the DNA of other cells. Only carcinogens and viruses are able to directly alter DNA. Our cells have internal defense mechanisms (antioxidants and DNA repair mechanisms) to combat and prevent this kind of DNA damage.

For cord blood, tissue rejection (graft versus host disease) is very minimal, and mismatches are well tolerated. That being said, the current consensus is that cord blood should be 4/6 HLA (human leukocyte antigens) matching.

How Are the Stem Cells Expanded?

And other related questions: You mentioned that stem cells are expanded in the laboratory in vitro? How many cell passages do the cells go through, and what tests are performed to ensure that the cells are homogeneous and retain their characteristics as primary totipotent stem cells vs getting transformed in vitro? How is this tested?

Answer: They are not expanded. They are basically tested, quarantined, washed, rinsed, counted, frozen.

Once Injected in the Body, Are Stem Cells Cleared from the Body?

And other related questions: You mentioned that the stem cells are cleared after eight months. Where do they reside? If cells were to lyse during normal wear and tear, have you seen any cases of autoantibody generation and autoimmunity on your follow-up with patients?

Answer: The cells attach to damaged areas through ligand bonding. Once locked in place, they secrete their own growth factors called secretomes to attract the bodies healing factors as well, create a daughter cell, and then, based on the frequency orientation of the cell to which they locked, to become that cell. There are no clearing factors. These are cells that will survive their lifespan. It is not a medication that is used of and then disappears. Wear and tear on any cell does cause lyses, but there would be no antibody generation because, again, the cells are not viewed as foreign. In my clinic, we have seen no such reactions.

Are There Some Patients Who Did Not Respond?

And other related questions: You indicated that in a small number of patients who did not respond, this was due to vascular insufficiency. How was this established?

Answer: Optimizing the body condition is always a plus. That can include increased vascular flow. I would not say we have assessed that is the reason for failure, as there are too many factors to measure. I, personally, would inject and begin nutrition simultaneously, and then decide on future injections at three to six months. This is why I created the Stem Cell Enhancement Program, so your potential for success is higher.

How Many Adverse Events Have Been Observed with Patients Receiving Cell Therapy from This Particular Institution That Is Supplying the Cells?

Answer: Since the procedure is noninvasive and relatively simple, side effects are seen only occasionally in a very small percentage of patients. **From our lab:** No adverse events have occurred at my office with the exception of flu-like symptoms with a sulpha patient. If a minor flu-like reaction occurs, it only lasts for twenty-four to forty-eight hours maximum. In fact, when this happens, it is a sign that the stem cells' anti-inflammatory properties are doing what they are supposed to.

What Is the Number of Sites of Injection and Cell Dosing?

And other related questions: You discussed number of sites of injection. We would like to understand the cell dosing per injection, since the responsiveness with most stem cells has an inverted U-type of response.

Answer: Dosing is going to be decided by our medical staff, reviewing protocols and guidelines from experienced advisors on size of joint, severity of problem, and multiplicity of locations. Therefore, it is purely a preference of the clinic. We have doctors doing .25 in each knee and some doing 1 cc in each knee with great results.

I Am Curious about the Laboratory That Supplies Your Cord Tissue MSCs for Injection.

And other related questions: What is the name of the manufacturer? Did they provide a package insert or certificate of analysis with or in advance of shipping the product? Can you share it with me? How do you store the cells prior to infusion?

Answer: Yes, we do utilize a few sources for our products, and we definitely control the specifications for the products, which is how we oversee and provide high-level quality products, regardless of the originating source. While we are a "third party," we do control the specifications, and we don't accept any that fall outside those requirements. Predictive Biotech is currently our preferred human umbilical cord tissue vendor. We have a certificate of analysis, and each batch has an analysis that is available on request, through us, our medical team at Regen Medicine.

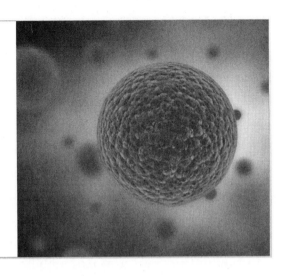

Is There Clinical Research?

A search of www.clinicaltrials.gov provides information on more than 5300 clinical trials being conducted worldwide

Where Can the Research on Stem Cells Be Found?

Answer: The scientific studies, research, and clinical trials on stem cell therapy is widely available from a variety of sources. As well, the resources in this book cite specific studies and provide a jumping-off point. Other places to find research papers and medical journals about stem cell studies include the following:

- International Journal of Stem Cells:
  http://www.ijstemcell.com/main.html

- Research Gate:
  https://www.researchgate.net/journal/1876-7753_Stem_Cell_Research

- U.S. National Library of Medicine:
  https://www.ncbi.nlm.nih.gov/pubmed/

- Regenerative Medicine Journal:
  https://www.futuremedicine.com/loi/rme

- OMICS International:
  https://www.omicsonline.org/scientific-journals.php

Why Are Stem Cells Controversial?

Answer: Stem cells are controversial because of their use in cloning. Although that use is completely different from the stem cell therapy we provide, cloning has put a damper on stem cell research as both sides argue the morality and ethics.

The other reason the use of stem cells for medical purposes is controversial is because of the use of stem cells from human embryos. This practice is frowned upon by many individuals, and since not everyone is aware of the different types of stem cell therapy, the controversy continues.

In our practice, we use *only* umbilical cord stem cells, so this controversy is not relevant to what we are doing.

Why We Choose Human Umbilical Cord Cells

Answer: The stem cells we use are from human umbilical cord blood. It is extracted from healthy, live, umbilical cord after it has been separated from mother and child.

The reasons we choose this type of stem cells fall into a few different categories:

1. **Sustainability:** This is a product of every birth, and is often discarded. There are new umbilical cords being thrown away daily.
2. **Young:** Umbilical cord blood contains a high number of young stem cells, ideal for the regeneration and anti-inflammatory effects required.
3. **Ethical:** There is no risk or uncertainty in the source of these stem cells, and the entire process is rigorously regulated from start to finish.

4. **Science-backed:** More and more research points to umbilical cord stem cells as having significant positive results for a multitude of patients.

Janice's Story—Needed Proof

"What makes my story so different is how against stem cells I was. Some of my friends called me an activist, but I was very vocal about the detrimental, ethical questions when blood cells are taken from humans, especially when they are too young to object. The image of stem cells connected to abortion, profiting from dead babies, as I called it, made it sick.

"I didn't learn until later, of course, that there are many different types of stem cell therapies, just as there are different sources of stem cells. It actually taught me a lot, just about researching things before speaking about them.

"It really humbles me, as so many people pointed out, I was contradicting myself. For so many years, I spread a message of lies. Then, it was like I had a transformation. And for the people closest to me, it seemed like I was a hypocrite.

"Eventually though, even they could not deny the improvement stem cell therapy made in my life. Finally, it felt like I was regaining control over my body, over the pain and weakness that I felt had kept me from enjoying life altogether.

"Cooking used to be my favorite thing, but arthritis and crippling pain kept me from creating any meals. Opening a container of food was as far as I got, and even then, more often than not, it

was take-out. Eating poorly and not moving much added to my feeling unwell.

"When a neighbor, one of the few people who still visited me, told me about stem cell therapy, I told her off. There was nothing worse than someone pretending to care about you, but really, they just want to be the first with the story of what is going on with you.

"Unfortunately, I couldn't wrap my head around someone wanting to help me. In my mind, she was trying to get rid of me, and I did not trust anyone. At the same time, I needed something to improve.

"Looking back, I really think my mental health was being affected by the physical pain. Just as I was about to give up and was seriously considering taking all of my pain pills at once, I saw an article called the 'Science and Safety of Stem Cells.'

"At the time, it was like a personal message or a slap in the face telling me to wake up. I read it, and then contacted the company it came from. It had to be a scam, I thought.

"The minute I spoke to someone at the office, my mind was put to ease. Everything was well laid out, and it was like the exact opposite of what I had been expecting. Their professional mannerisms were warm and welcoming, and they were not made nervous by my probing questions.

"After that first meeting, I went from skeptic to booking an appointment. And I was beginning to realize how deep things could get when you are only focused on one aspect of things. People who are vocal against something need to have the science to back up their claims, at least, that is my two cents.

"I didn't, and now I was walking proof that I was a hypocrite. That was fine with me though, because I was walking again, and that was all that mattered. I could get up and spend my day doing this and that.

"As well, I could work again, which was a relief financially, but it also gave me purpose. I just hope other people open themselves up to the new science. It can be hard because we hear things and then we assume, but when we take time to try to understand, it becomes more and more clear.

"The only thing I would do differently is go for it sooner. I think it would have been even more beneficial if I could have had stem cell therapy before the pain became so severe."

Ethics and Laws

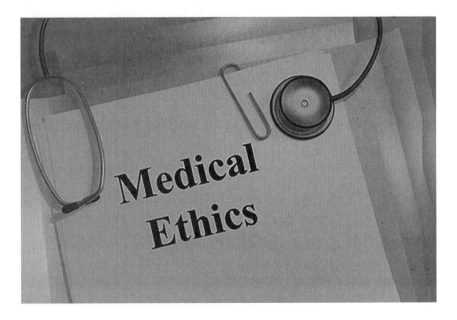

The science of stem cells is going to continue, as the therapeutic and biological potential is just beginning to be understood. Although ethical issues abound, especially in regard to embryonic and fetal stem cells, more and more research and investigation is being completed in order to maintain a safe environment for all involved.

The evidence is mounting that:

> . . . *stem cells recovered postnatal from the umbilical cord, including the umbilical cord blood cells, amnion/placenta, umbilical cord vein, or umbilical cord matrix cells, are a readily available and inexpensive source of cells that are capable of forming many different cell types (i.e., they are "multipotent").*

Following the science and the studies leads us to the confidence in the procedure and process of stem cell therapy. The ethical issues that exist can be separated based on the source of the stem cells and whether there are other oversights in place.

In the United States, the Food and Drug Administration (FDA), monitors and regulates medical procedures and therapies. As such, they have comprised a set of guidelines and requirements to prevent potential risk.

According to the Commissioner of the FDA, continued investigation into the safety of stem cell therapy is something they are committed to. In a statement, the agency emphasizes its regulatory process:

> We understand that there will be questions, and it will take time for product developers to determine whether their products require FDA approval. Our policy will allow product manufacturers that time to engage with the FDA to determine if they need to submit a marketing authorization application and, if so, seek guidance on how to submit their application to the FDA for approval.

To be clear, we remain committed to ensuring that patients have access to safe and effective regenerative medicine products as efficiently as possible. We are also committed to making sure we take action against products being unlawfully marketed that pose a potential significant risk to their safety. The framework we're announcing today gives us the solid platform we need to continue to take enforcement action against a small number of clearly unscrupulous actors.

With this balanced approach, we're well positioned to support and help advance breakthrough science, like regenerative medicine, and promote responsible and flexible regulation that leverages science to advance public health.

-GIOKAS ET AL. THE ROLE OF HLA IN CORD BLOOD
TRANSPLANTATION. BONE MARROW RES. 2012

CHAPTER 7
Is Stem Cell
Therapy for You?

Know Your Health

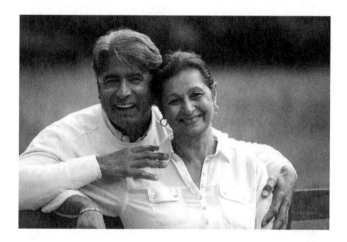

The intent of this book is to help you take a deep breath and learn about how stem cell therapy can improve your health. As well, we want to encourage you to take control of your journey to wellness. Whether you are looking to reduce inflammation, improve your immune system, or get a handle on areas of pain in your life, stem cell therapy is worth your consideration.

When you think about your health, you might say, "Yeah, it bothers me, but it is not horrible; it is manageable." Based on how you feel right now, you might have your condition under control, whether or not your symptoms are caused by the following:

- Joint stiffness or injury
- Degenerative issues
- Autoimmune disorder
- Neurological damage
- Tissue damage
- Chronic pain
- Inflammation
- Arthritis
- Cardiovascular Issues
- Spinal cord injury

Now, all of these are long-term issues. Imagine, if you will, how you will feel given another five, ten, or twenty years. Chances are, because of your current condition, your health could gradually decline into further pain and suffering, and your quality of life would suffer. So many people spend the last decade of their lives this way, and it is sad, because it does not have to happen for most people.

Be honest with your understanding about your own health, so you can avoid that undesirable end. If there is any chance at all that you may end up becoming a burden on your family and friends, and losing your freedom to declining health, look now into what can be done about it. The future of your health is in your hands.

Stem cell therapy is one of the newest options available in regenerative medicine. It is being used for a wide range of conditions, and the research continues to expand every year. As more and more patients are seeing their lives changed through the regenerative properties of stem cells, the science is backing their stories.

Now that governments, health-care organizations, and medical education institutes are taking steps to further stem cell research, it is becoming more and more available. As well, the regulation and oversight are making it safer than ever. It was just a matter, all along, of the mainstream health and wellness industry catching up with all of the scientific breakthroughs in so many varied health conditions.

Seeing the facts and hearing people speak about their own experiences brings hope and relief to so many patients. Once they understand the process and how minimally invasive of a procedure it is, they can see how it fits right into the picture they have of their health.

So if something is causing you discomfort in your life now, you can be sure that in another few years, it will only get worse.

Ask yourself the following questions:

1. At what point is it going to become unbearable?
2. How is it affecting my loved ones?
3. Do I have the resources to get additional help as my body weakens?
4. How many years do I have left?
5. What am I really missing out on in my life?

The answer to these questions is different for everyone. The one thing most people have in common is that they do not want to find out just how bad it can get.

No one intentionally choses a less-than-optimal life. In the same way, no one chooses to miss out on being involved in their grandchildren's lives. Instead of giving up your favorite activities and doing what makes you happy, it is time to take a look at all your options.

If you had the choice, would you rather follow conventional wisdom and slowly decline or be willing to try something that may be new, but is also tried-and-true?

Would you rather:

- Stay on your medication and wait and see, or give your natural healing a boost?
- Have surgery to replace a body part, or encourage regeneration through stem cells?
- Take whatever treatment insurance covers, or try something different that might change your life?
- Watch from the sidelines consumed with pain and discomfort, or participate and feel joy in all aspects of your life?
- Go on one last vacation, or try a procedure that could give you your life back?
- Be isolated and in pain, or checking things off your bucket list?
- Count down the hours until your next pill, or enjoy the rich abundance the world has to offer?
- Leave your health in the hands of people who have stopped looking for answers, or find a path to regenerative healing?
- Watch the minutes tick by as you are handicapped by your condition, or take a breath at the end of the day wondering how it went by so fast?

It is your life and your choice. Your health is in your hands. Only you know your health, and only you can decide what path your wellness journey can take. I can help you with information, medical knowledge, and experience, but how and what happens is totally up to you.

So let's remember the contents of this book with a thought to the individual healing process that each individual is undertaking. Stem cell therapy is an option that is changing lives, but the first step is being informed. Knowing the different types of therapies and sources of stem cells makes sure you can choose the one that is likely to have the most positive results.

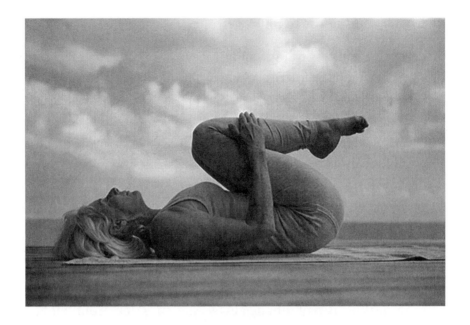

When umbilical cord stem cells are used, this therapy is an ethical, safe, and regulated option to encourage healing and regeneration throughout your body. It is a noninvasive, drug-free procedure that begins reducing inflammation and pain at the source. Since it provides multiple benefits that work in conjunction with the body's natural healing process, research continues to move toward stem cell therapy.

As regulation begins to align with the research and development, stem cell therapy is now becoming an option for more patients across the country and the world. We are finally catching up on what athletes have been using for more than a decade.

*"Knowing your health means knowing
all options available to restore it."*

Don't let your health decline another day before you take steps to improve your condition. Too often, we are willing to accept less for ourselves, when we should be only willing to accept better.

So YOU can choose to improve your:

- Body's natural healing ability
- Knee and joint stiffness
- Energy level
- Chronic pain
- Level and quality of sleep
- Outlook on life
- Belief in the power of your body
- Knowledge of regenerative health care

After all, you only get one body and so such time to enjoy your life. It all starts with your choice to want something different for yourself and to be willing to get it, instead of following the current system.

Your healing is not financially viable in a for-profit medical system. Keeping you paying for prescriptions, surgery, and short-term treatments ensures repeat visits to doctors, and more money in their pockets.

So often we do not want to think about the callousness and corruption. Fair enough, because that will get anyone feeling down. But don't allow yourself to succumb to the belief in a system that wants your money.

All we ask is that you follow the science and the understanding of your own health and body. Scientists are finding, repeatedly, that stem cells promote regeneration and healing, as well as reduce inflammation in many different locations all over the body.

Human Stem Cell Applications

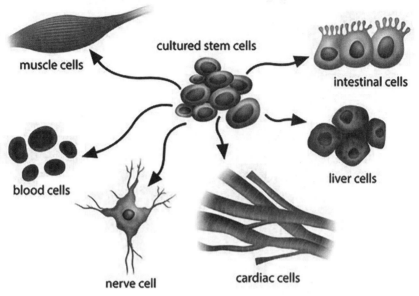

muscle cells

cultured stem cells

intestinal cells

blood cells

liver cells

nerve cell

cardiac cells

Sandra's Story—Autoimmune Disease

"My husband and I were planning our last cruise. All our friends were coming, but it was starting to feel like a living funeral. It was time to face facts as my autoimmune disease was wreaking havoc on my day-to-day life. I spent a lot of the time resting and exhausted, and my body was not functioning; everything was a struggle.

"A few years earlier, I was the life of the party. We had a group of friends we traveled with a couple of times a year, and we all got together often. Usually they came to our house, and I made five-course meals for them. I loved to be the hostess and see a beautiful evening come together.

"As time went on, it took more effort to do anything, and a supper like that took three days to recover from. I chalked it up to getting older. Then, I was diagnosed with a thyroid condition and arthritis, back-to-back. Medication for one would make symptoms of the other worse.

"Now our social life was not fun any longer. It was work, and I dreaded our get togethers. We had declined the previous trip, and it was the first time we missed one. I had a reaction to a recent medication and was hospitalized. I told my husband to go without me and, of course, he refused. Then I got what the doctors called the flu, and what I remember as the sickness of my life.

"After that, I seemed to decline very quickly. No matter what I tried, I got worse and worse. So I told my husband we needed to go on one last cruise, while I still could. He was not supportive, at first; he said it was like I was planning my funeral.

"Still, I spoke with some friends, and they agreed to help, and we began to plan my last vacation. While this happened, my husband, who had unwillingly agreed to the trip, was going behind my back. During his spare time, and when I was not around, he was searching for any alternative health option that might help me.

"Even if I had given up hope, he wasn't ready to yet. And so, that is how I came across stem cell therapy. One night, when I was soaking in the tub, the one place I could feel some relief, he came and told me we needed to talk.

"It was odd because he was usually the strong, silent type and was much more casual in conversation. I couldn't remember

him ever sounding so serious, and I was, frankly, a little worried. By the time I dried off and joined him in the kitchen, I assumed the worst.

"Now I remember it like it was yesterday because I was wrapping my hair in a towel as I entered the kitchen, and my husband was sitting at the kitchen table with folders and pamphlets in front of him. He had notes and looked ready to give a presentation.

"Maybe that is not the weirdest thing for some people, but for me it was like a switch—from my life before to my life after. This was the moment where everything changed for the better.

"He sat me down and told me what he learned about stem cell therapy, including people we both knew who had seen positive results. It was eye-opening for me, and I admit I felt a little embarrassed that I hadn't been looking for a solution. But everyone had told me there was no solution.

"Everything made sense, and I was actually able to receive the stem cell therapy before our big trip. We went away a month after, and it was like I was back. My energy levels had increased, and I was able to keep up and enjoy my time with everyone.

"I feel so blessed and thank the doctors and the health-care team and, of course, my husband for pushing me into it. They have all been so wonderfully positive it has inspired my new journey in life."

What Do Stem Cells Do?

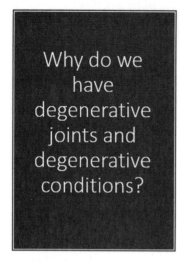

Why do we have degenerative joints and degenerative conditions?

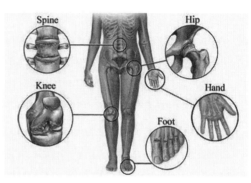

The most important thing to focus on with stem cells is also the reason they were discovered. Stem cells are different from other types of cells because they can differentiate, regenerating into different types of cells depending on what is needed.

The illustration shows so concisely how stem cells can be used in such a wide variety of ways. Everyone has stem cells that originate in different areas of the body. As we age, some stem cells die off while all our cells get older.

Then as we injure ourselves, or have illnesses and other trauma, our natural regenerative ability lessens. With stem cell therapy, the procedure provides assistance to the bone, cartilage, tissue, and other systems in the body that need it.

As the research matches the feedback from patients seeing amazing results, stem cell therapy is being opened up to more complex and varied conditions and situations. Finding the adaptability of umbilical cord stem cells has provided a safe means to continue in this way.

Encourage the Body's Own Natural Healing

Our body has systems in place to heal and regenerate. It also has the ability to send messages when something is not going right. Instead of masking these messages with medication or cutting them off via surgery, we must learn from them and use them in an effort to move toward good health.

By encouraging natural healing, you can learn the information required to know whether stem cell therapy might be the right choice for you. The best way to start yourself on a healthy path is to find out how you can improve your overall wellness.

So often we forget about how amazing our bodies are, and overlook the major ways we heal ourselves. Just a few of the long list of types of natural regeneration that takes place in our own bodies gives us an idea of how stem cell therapy can accentuate that process:

- Blood clotting to protect a wound while the skin regrows
- Regrow of hair and nails
- Broken bones re-fusing together
- The rejuvenating power of sleep
- Natural immunity to the bacteria in our environment
- White blood cells and their germ-fighting antibodies
- The mucous and fluid in the eyes, nose, and other systems that protect and heal the body's systems.
- Love: many studies have shown the healing power of love and emotional connection
- Inflammation (as a side note, we have talked about the negative effects of inflammation throughout this book, but it is actually a process designed to protect and heal the body).
- The liver can regrow when a portion is removed or damaged, and it can also compensate for the gallbladder.
- Stomach cells regrow around every four days as the acid eats away at the lining so quickly.

The purpose of this book, including the stories of the patients with whom I have had the privilege of working, is to serve as a guide to those of you still searching for answers. If any of their stories resonate with you, take it as a sign that you, too, could see the positive results they did. It is about bringing hope through knowledge to people who are looking for a change for the better.

A Tale of Two Twins

"My sister, Megan, was always the healthy sister. She was fit and athletic, and she ate healthy food. Now, I wasn't overly unhealthy. I didn't go out of my way to harm my body, but I was a bit clumsy, uncoordinated, and frankly, I would rather sit on the couch and have coffee and a chat with someone.

"Growing up, neither of us had any major health concerns, which means we took our health for granted. As we grew into adulthood, I was starting to realize I couldn't just eat whatever I wanted anymore.

"One day, my sister was over for coffee; she had biked over from across town, and I was still in my pajamas. She was talking about work and some other projects that were going on, and I just saw how bright and full of life she was.

"For some reason, on that day, it struck me, and the thought would not go away. As sisters, twins even, why did she have so much vitality, and I was always exhausted and lagging behind. I had never experienced the joyful bursts of energy and excitements the way my sister did.

"Everything always seemed to take me longer and cause more aches and pains throughout my body. Instead of trying to get better, I was spending time trying to figure out where all my sister's energy came from.

"When I talked to my doctor about it, he ran some tests and discovered I had Hashimoto's and likely my thyroid issues were the cause of most of my symptoms. I was ecstatic. This, I thought, would be the end of all my problems.

"I expected the doctor would write me a prescription, I would take it, feel amazing, and get on with my life, thank you very much. Sad to say, that didn't happen. For so long, I held out hope, but my symptoms got worse.

"Now everyone seemed to act like it was all in my head, and I was even more tired and frustrated than ever before. I started to distance myself from my family because I felt like I was dragging everyone down with me.

"Desperate for something different for a change, I came across stem cell therapy and attended an initial consult. Right away, I booked the procedure, but then a strange thing happened. Everyone I told about it tried to talk me out of it, claiming things like it was too dangerous or it wouldn't help anyway.

"I have to say, it raised some doubts. So I went back to my notes and the literature I was given and I reassured myself that it was not only safe, it was likely the best option for me. So my appointment came and went, and it was a completely noninvasive and an overly professional experience. That's not the strange part though. Almost immediately after the appointment, I started to feel better. My energy was improving by the minute, it seemed.

"As people saw my healing process occur, they would ask me what my secret was. For some of them, I got a little cheeky. I responded that they didn't want to hear about stem cell therapy before, so why would they want to hear about it now.

"The really strange part was that my sister got hurt at almost the exact same time. She had fallen off her bike and twisted her knee. It was difficult for her to walk, so her activity level slowed right down. And she wasn't getting any better.

"Her doctors said she would be lucky if she could see gradual improvement sometime, but couldn't promise anything. So she and I switched places as she was there, in front of the TV on the couch, and I biked over to see her.

"When I mentioned my sister at my six-week, follow-up appointment, the clinic suggested that she come for a consultation. It surprised me because I did not know that this procedure was beneficial for knee pain or injury.

"It was like, well you learn something new every day! My sister was dubious too. She couldn't believe there was some miracle cure that would fix both of us. But since I had tried it and lived, she figured she could give it a shot.

"As she regained movement and mobility, the results were unanimous. Both of us were in so much better shape after stem cell therapy, and we believe the procedure worked better than expected.

"Now my sister and I are biking together. We have both worked hard on our healing journey. The one thing I learned, throughout it all, was how stem cell therapy can help people with such vastly different health issues."

The Act of Regeneration

Since stem cells have been discovered, when used in therapy, their most remarkable and adaptable aspect is that stem cells are attracted to areas of inflammation or those in need of repair and regeneration. If one of my patients comes in with joint pain, we can target the exact area that the degenerative condition is wreaking havoc on the body.

Sometimes our bodies need a boost, especially if they have been repairing issues and conditions over a long period of time. As those cells get worn and ragged, the body is much slower to respond to the call for regeneration.

We seek to provide, through education about stem cell therapy, an understanding of the balance of degeneration and regeneration and what that means to your health. When inflammation in a specific area occurs, the loss of cellular function in the area is the result. To ensure ongoing rebuilding of tissues in the body, ample regenerative properties are required. Stem cell therapy works with your body to fulfill those rejuvenating requirements.

As degenerative issues ebb and flow based on life changes and regenerative availability, our body is always working toward a natural rhythm.

"Inflammation is like the body's alarm system
that something is out of rhythm."

Both regeneration and degeneration naturally occur, depending on what stage in the body's cycles they are occurring in. In some cases, the inflammation is integral in the healing process.

Unfortunately, when there is no balance, the overall health of the body goes into a state of degeneration. And when left unchecked, degeneration can advance and develop into some pretty difficult-to-repair, ongoing situations.

When regeneration is no longer sustainable, fatal diseases in many different areas are often the result. Some of them are as follows:

- Cardiovascular disease
- Pulmonary disease like COPD
- Alzheimer's
- Thyroid disease
- Diabetes
- Arthritis
- Muscular dystrophy
- Autoimmune disease
- Cystic fibrosis (CF)

As degeneration is ramped up to an out-of-control level by the ongoing inflammation, it is enough to give anyone a feeling of uncertainty in the unknown. Still, the goal is to reduce the levels of stress and strain on the body.

Stress has a major impact on how the body heals itself. Certain lifestyle aspects influence how we manage stress through the following:

- Sleep schedule
- Diet and nutrients
- Lifestyle and recreation
- Emotional well-being
- Work/Life balance
- Environmental toxins

Even in the most severe health issues, the patient usually retains some control over the outcome. Even if you have a debilitating condition caused by degeneration, you can see improvement and encourage regeneration.

If you ask yourself some specific questions, you will clearly build upon your understanding as to the regeneration process. Sometimes what seems like the smallest detail or situation can be improved upon.

1. When I sleep, is my body resting and recovering?
2. Do I have a difficult time going to bed or falling asleep?
3. Have I noticed an increase in emotional stress?
4. Are the people in my life positively or negatively impacting me?
5. Can I make my surrounding environment healthier?
6. Where do I feel the most weakness, pain, or discomfort?
7. When I am worried or stressed, do I notice an increase in symptoms?

In order to get a better picture of where and how a degenerative condition is progressing, we spend a lot of time offering advice and assistance to those whose bodies cannot keep up with the ill effects of their conditions.

As we age, the regeneration process becomes limited. Our bodies all eventually die; stem cell therapy seeks to prolong this process. Since our stem cells are naturally depleted over time, the body often needs a repair mechanism much beyond our current capabilities.

The Angry Widow

"When I went to the doctor, I intended to be as angry as possible. If stem cells were so wonderful, why didn't they save my husband? He wasn't even offered it as an option; instead, they just let him die.

"His death angered me alright, but it shook everything I thought I knew about the world. I thought doctors learned unbiased and scientific information regarding health and healing. I thought foreign influences would not affect our basic right to health. I was mistaken and got to learn devastating info about the medical system, firsthand.

"So why weren't the doctors able to help my husband? When he died, I lost everything. It felt like the air had been taken out of my sails; I was devastated. He had been my pillar for so many years, and I felt lost without him. I also felt cheated that he had disappeared before my eyes in less than a year.

"When he was diagnosed with ALS, I didn't have a clue that meant we would lose him so quickly. Nine months later, his body had shut down, and he was gone. Life was a blur after that, because everything we had planned, everything we had, and everything we did was together.

"Dan and I were a team, and even our children couldn't cheer me up; they just reminded me of what I lost and what we would all be missing without him in our lives. Obviously, at that time, I didn't even stop to consider my health at all. My body was recovering from the shock of losing my husband, and it began spiralling out of control.

"It started with a thyroid issue, which the doctors figured was caused by all the stress I was under. I was gaining weight and felt sick all the time, and I didn't care. My breathing was getting heavier, and it seemed like every day I found some new problem.

"After a while I stopped trying at all and kept myself in my house. Through my new computer that the kids bought to keep in touch with me, I found online shopping, and I ordered everything I needed.

"But I didn't keep in touch with my kids. I didn't respond to their silly jokes, I did not answer their heartfelt messages, and I did not comment on the pictures they sent me of my beautiful grandchildren. It hurt too much, and I didn't want to let go and move on because it felt like moving away from my husband.

"Finally, when my daughter had not heard from me, she showed up unannounced, and she was pissed off. She told me I was being selfish and lazy. Then, she talked about everything that I was missing out on.

"It is true, I tried to tune her out. I ignored her and I acted like a two-year-old and covered my head to pretend she wasn't there. What can I say, I was desperate? But then she said something I have never forgotten.

"'Dad would hate to see you like this.'

"That was a wakeup call I was not ready for. She was right; my husband would never want me to waste my life feeling sorry for myself, and he told me exactly that. He wanted me to live life to the fullest.

"So I cried, and I hugged her and I said I was sorry. That night I stayed up, straightened up, and got my house in order. I couldn't believe it had gotten so bad. And yet I couldn't sleep. My health was poor because I had been ignoring it for so long, but during all that time, I had a niggling feeling that going to the doctor was useless.

"In part, I think it was because of how my husband died; I no longer trusted doctors, so hearing from them about my own condition was quite traumatizing. As well, it almost felt like I had an underlying knowledge that health was more complicated than just treating the symptoms.

"Certainly, I did not want to waste away like my husband, but I did not want to be reliant on medication or have to go through surgery either. There had to be a better way, and I became determined to find it.

"And with most great things, I found the solutions right under my nose. Stem cell therapy changed me from an angry widow to a joyful grandma living life to the fullest. And for that I am truly thankful."

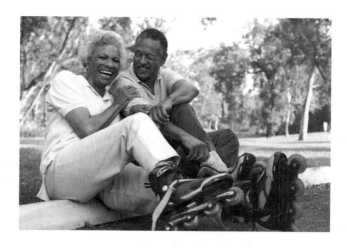

Aging Gracefully

As you age, your body naturally heals more slowly. Certain processes and systems begin to slow down also. Although some signs of aging are obvious, others are slower to become noticeable.

The body's processes reach a peak as we mature, and then begin to decline. Different areas of the body age in different ways:

Cells: Overall, as we age, cellular function starts to decline. Since cells can only divide a certain number of times, they eventually reach an end. Aging cells affect all other body systems.

Organs: Over time, our organs start to function less optimally; however, in many cases such as the brain and heart, lifestyle practices and exercises can slow or prevent the effects of aging in these organs.

Bones and Tendons: Both bones and tendons, especially in the major joints, become weakened over time. Certain conditions like osteoporosis can speed up this process. As well, changes in the fluid that protects bones and tendons can cause increased wear and tear.

Muscles: After the age of thirty, muscles begin to slowly decline. This is partly due to the decreasing level of growth-hormone production. For muscles, exercise, or the lack thereof, will either accelerate or slow down this process.

Eyes: As people age, the different areas of the eye, including the lens, pupil, and nerves become less effective, mostly due to overuse.

Blood Vessels: During the aging process, partly due to lifestyle choices, blood vessels become stiff and less effective. Blood pressure often increases, as arteries are not able to expand as well as they used to.

To age gracefully, your health and wellness needs must be balanced. For some people, stem cell therapy is the kick-start they need for a rejuvenated life journey. Maintaining health and reversing certain signs of aging are already the natural tendency of stem cells.

The image below shows how bone mass deceases with age, in both men and women. It is significant to note, that after age forty, our bodies start to go through rapid bone loss up until age sixty. This affects how the body naturally heals and where stem cells can greatly improve your chances of healing.

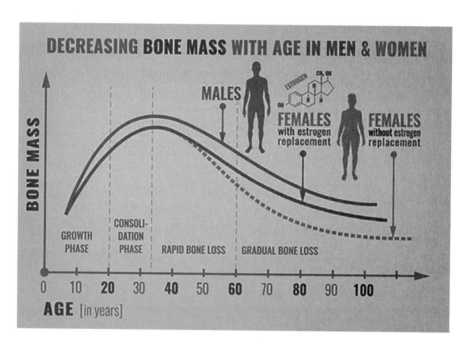

258

The Belaney Family

"*Even though I am telling you my story, it doesn't start with me, not even close. While I was out of the country, on assignment, my family was going through a crisis. The thing is I didn't even find out about this until later. They didn't want to worry me.*

"*The first person in my family who had stem cell therapy was my father. He is the most stubborn and private man you have ever met. So, no one even knew about it until much later when the crisis came to a head.*

"*We have a close family, and yet we try too hard to protect each other. When our mom died not long after my youngest sister was born, we made a pact to always stay together. There were ten children in all, and I am the second oldest.*

"*My older brother was always right beside my dad. When mom died, he stepped in to make sure all the younger kids got where they were supposed to, and he was there for all of us while my dad continued to work and support us.*

"*As each sibling finished school and got a job, almost all of us settled nearby and met up for Sunday supper together, or if not, we were all together for the holidays. No matter what.*

"*Eventually though, for most of us, there were times when we couldn't make it. Like all the times I was on assignment, overseas. It wasn't really funny, but it worked, and we were making it work. Each sibling has their own children as well, so that makes for a big family.*

"*Well, about a month after my dad had surgery, my nephew became ill. At first, it looked like a flu, but run the numbers and you will see it was huge. His condition got worse and worse until enough was enough.*

"First, it was my nephew, and then his dad, my brother. Then, my sister, who held our family together, became very sick and no one could help her.

"Angrily, my dad let the cat out of the bag, Each and every one of us has since gotten stem cell therapy. It happened so fast. After the truth about stem cell therapies was looked at, each of us had a little project where we would seek out the help of others.

"In total, five of us received stem cell therapy for five different issues all around the same time. It was remarkable to us how this option brought us back from desperation to hope."

Is Stem Cell Therapy for You?

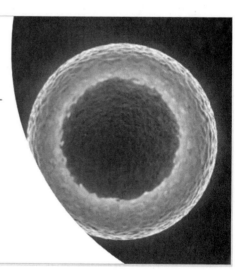

Stem Cell Therapy

- Direction healthcare is headed
- Used by athlete's for 10+ years
- Changes in rules & regulations have allowed stem cell therapy to be available at reasonable cost

There is only one person who knows whether stem cell therapy is the next step for you—and that is you. By reading this book and pursuing the resources we have discussed, you can now make that decision with confidence.

Keep this book close by as you make decisions about your health and journey to wellness. Review the information, especially as it relates specifically to your condition, so that you can move forward and live a life that frees you of the constrictions of your ill-health.

It is your health, and your choice what you want to do with this beautiful life you have been given. All I ask is that you be honest with yourself in what you want for your future. Sometimes the biggest steps toward a better life are so tiny, you might miss them.

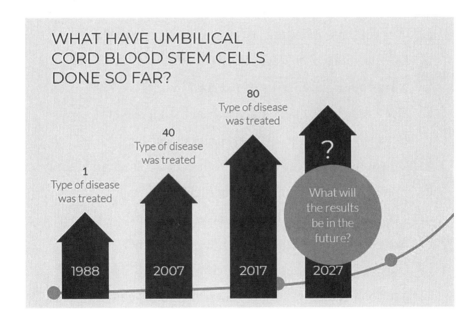

WHAT HAVE UMBILICAL CORD BLOOD STEM CELLS DONE SO FAR?

80
Type of disease was treated

40
Type of disease was treated

1
Type of disease was treated

?
What will the results be in the future?

1988   2007   2017   2027

IS STEM CELL THERAPY FOR YOU? A CHECKLIST

☐ Do you have a long-term health problem or chronic condition?

☐ Do you have an autoimmune disorder?

☐ Have you tried medication or surgery?

☐ Are your joints stiff and sore?

☐ Is it more difficult to get up in the morning?

☐ Do you have a hard time sleeping?

☐ When you walk, do your knees buckle or legs feel weak?

☐ Are you able to breathe and eat without pain?

☐ Do you have back pain?

☐ Have you ever felt low energy even after resting?

☐ Can you remember the last time you felt great?

☐ Do you suffer from degenerative issues?

☐ Have you experienced a spinal cord injury?

☐ Does your body take longer to heal than it used to?

☐ Have you noticed an increase in illnesses?

☐ Do you want to keep up with your active friends and family?

☐ Are you looking for a pain-free life?

☐ Can you remember the last time you felt well?

☐ Are you avoiding activities you used to enjoy?

☐ Do you feel powerless to your condition?

☐ Are you tired of waiting for doctors who have no answers?

☐ Have you started seeking alternative healing processes?

If you answered yes to four or more questions, you likely have a similar story to many of our patients and would do well in seeking more information.

A consultation will determine what you likely already know, stem cell therapy could just be the beginning of a wonderful new health journey for you.

As you progress on your journey to health, keep up the good work and keep fighting for something better. Be prepared to ask questions, look at the research and know how your body's healing systems naturally work.

It is my intention in writing this book to help you gain the knowledge you need to move forward. It is the same intention I have with all my patients and the people with whom I speak about wellness. Be empowered with this knowledge and use it to ensure you get the best possible health care that fits your condition and unique circumstances.

Study the information about your specific situation and investigate the science of how it all works. Also talk about it to friends, family, and your health-care providers. You are sure to get mixed reactions, but you might be surprised. The important thing is do your own research and focus on the facts. You only have one shot at your health, so take the time to find out how to boost your vitality and enjoy your life to the fullest.

Now that we all know better, we can do better for ourselves, for our patients, and for generations to come.

Stem Cell Enhancement Program

HOW TO GET EVEN BETTER RESULTS WITH YOUR STEM CELL THERAPY

Helping You Heal Faster

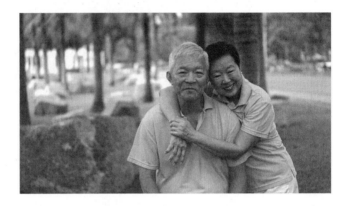

Sometimes struggling to find answers regarding our health is overwhelming. There is so much information to process. As well, as we have seen, so many different body systems contribute to and are affected by one condition or disease. That is why we take a whole-health approach with every patient we see.

We are offering our stem cell patients a complimentary, six-week, video enhancement program. If you have had stem cell injections, we want to give you the very best chance possible to not only heal, but to allow those stem cells to regenerate to their full potential. This is a free gift to our patients. For those people who may have received stem cell therapy at another clinic, we want to help you as well, and you are welcome to purchase the enhancement program through www.regenhealthmed.com.

Stem cell therapy does amazing things for people with a wide variety of health issues. But we do not just complete the procedure and send you on your way thinking, "Now what?"

I had one patient who came to see me while he was recovering from a failed back surgery. He had multiple health issues all connected to a spinal cord injury. After a six-hour surgery and a two-week hospital stay, he was discharged with no further advice or information. His discharge papers that usually should give detailed follow-up information on rest and recovery were blank.

Left on his own, his recovery didn't go well. Now this patient's story has a happy ending, and when he came to see us, we began a program tailored to helping him regain his health. The point is, we do not offer quick fixes, and we are here for you not just through your recovery period, but in the long run.

We want to support you through the whole process, so you can get the most out of the stem cells. This program is part of our office protocol for stem cell therapy, but we also offer it to patients who have received stem cells from another medical center.

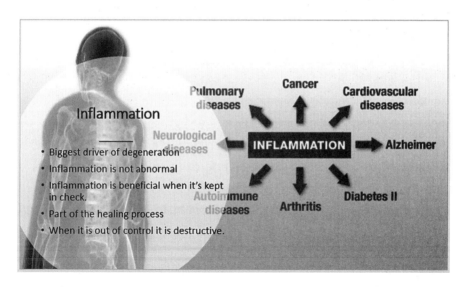

The Struggle with Inflammation

So many people are struggling with health issues, and they are not getting answers. Even after a diagnosis, people are not feeling any better. The fact is, we need to make the inflammation connection.

Often, patients are struggling with inflammation, and they don't even know it. The effects are catastrophic, and as a nation, even globally, we are not doing enough to educate, prevent, and treat the devastation that it causes.

Some of the scariest health statistics are related to inflammation, and most people do not realize it. I would go as far as to say that a huge majority of the causes of death in this country is connected to inflammation.

Look at just a few of the staggering statistics:

- The leading cause of death in America is cardiovascular disease with close to sixty-four million Americans suffering from some form. In 2001, almost one million people died from cardiovascular disease.
- In 2012, a study showed that nearly half of Americans suffer from a chronic disease.
- Seven of the ten top diseases in 2014 were chronic diseases.
- Eighty-six percent of health-care costs come from patients with chronic health issues.
- Fifty million Americans suffer from some type of allergy, and over the last two decades there has been a 100 percent increase in hay fever.

These numbers are continuing to rise and only show a fraction of the story. They show a glimpse into a scary truth. These are not random stats; they are all connected to inflammation.

The thing is, many of these are an autoimmune condition. Autoimmune-related inflammation occurs as a defense mechanism. When your body is injured, the immune system sends chemical messengers to the site to begin the healing process.

Then, when it goes awry, and the immune system turns against itself, one of many different conditions begins to develop. Looking at the sheer number of people struggling with inflammation, it becomes clear there is a serious health crisis unfolding.

These are some of the diseases and conditions that share underlying inflammation issues:

- Knee pain
- Shoulder pain
- Arthritis
- Parkinson's disease
- Autoimmune disease
- Cardiovascular disease
- COPD
- Diabetes
- Kidney function
- Spinal cord injury
- Skin trauma
- Stroke
- Brain injury

This list is just a handful of the hundreds of inflammatory diseases affecting people on a grand scale. Currently, most of these diseases and conditions are treated individually, and the connections are not often made, unless the patient is being seen by a more holistically minded medical team.

Inflammatory Diseases Share Some Similarities

Many of the life-threatening diseases and illnesses that we are told to watch for are inflammatory diseases. As we age, we often see signs or symptoms of these, sometimes fatal, diseases, and yet the connection is not often made that the issue is inflammation.

The health issues in the list above and many others that also stem from inflammation share some similarities. By looking at how they are related, we are better able to provide a healing program that works.

Inflammatory diseases share the following traits:

- **Chronic:** In many cases, fatal health conditions caused by inflammation are debilitating and worsen over time.
- **Incurable:** While many different treatments, medications, and surgical procedures are used to mitigate the symptoms and prolong a patient's health, inflammatory diseases do not have a cure.
- **Degeneration:** Inflammatory diseases attack and destroy cells and tissue in a particular area of the body. This is often made worse as we age, as the body is less able to defend itself and regenerate.
- **Increasing:** Every year, more and more people are being diagnosed with inflammatory diseases, even though public awareness campaigns and preventative measures are on the rise. Medical advancements are astonishing, and yet, the number of patients suffering also increases.

Though it is not all bad news. Understanding the inflammation connection has helped health-care providers like my clinic find new solutions. In fact, the commonality between all these conditions that we focus on is that stem cell therapy is improving the symptoms of inflammatory disease across the board. Every day, more patients are regaining their health and vitality instead of being stuck and bogged down in the symptoms of their disease.

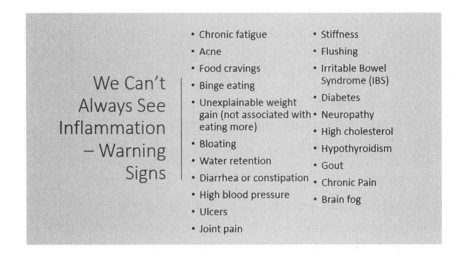

We Can't Always See Inflammation – Warning Signs

- Chronic fatigue
- Acne
- Food cravings
- Binge eating
- Unexplainable weight gain (not associated with eating more)
- Bloating
- Water retention
- Diarrhea or constipation
- High blood pressure
- Ulcers
- Joint pain
- Stiffness
- Flushing
- Irritable Bowel Syndrome (IBS)
- Diabetes
- Neuropathy
- High cholesterol
- Hypothyroidism
- Gout
- Chronic Pain
- Brain fog

One Solution for Hundreds of Conditions

Once we have made the connection and understand how stem cell therapy works to improve inflammatory disease, the question becomes: Why not help erase, reduce, and even reverse your risk for all these conditions (and many more) at the same time?

And why not take steps to improve the inflammatory epidemic, in just over a month?

Of course, doctors and medical professionals that profit from your illness don't want you to know what I am talking about. There is one solution for hundreds of diseases and conditions, and that is stem cell therapy with our enhancement program. Instead of masking the symptoms, it works to eliminate the root cause.

Which of these experiences would you like to do away with in your own life?

- Chronic pain leaving you immobile
- Chest tightness leaving you breathless
- Exhaustion from tossing and turning all night
- Weight gain regardless of diet or exercise

These outcomes and many more health improvements are things I see every day in my practice. Although it might seem remarkable, it is very likely the thing that is causing you the most suffering is doing so needlessly.

The thing is, the science backs up what I am saying here. Hundreds of studies and clinical trials have been conducted for years, and all of them show positive correlation between stem cell therapy and reduced inflammation.

A Two-Step Process to Healing and Regeneration

Countless treatments, medications, and procedures claim to be a quick fix or instant cure. We do not claim that. Aware of the natural healing and regeneration cycle of the human body, we emphasize a process designed to enhance the health outcomes.

STEP 1: Get stem cell injection therapy

Some stem cell clinics will simply provide you with an injection and then send you on your way. So for this step I am going to describe what happens in our office. I cannot speak for anywhere else, but for step one, our involvement goes way beyond the injection.

At the initial consult, if you decide that stem cell injection is something that might benefit you, we agree on the best day to accomplish this. Then, five days prior to the injections, we touch base with some recommendations on how to prepare for the procedure in order to see the most significant results.

STEP 2: Stem cell enhancement program—six-week curriculum

The stem cell enhancement program is a six-week curriculum that helps you stack everything in your favor. For this reason, that's why you will get my stem cell enhancement curriculum as a free bonus.

During this time, you will be guided on what to eat and what not to eat, the right stretches, and core exercises. You will receive specific nutrients that will help you regenerate faster. This step-by-step video program will give you the tools to help enhance the healing potential for the rest of your life. Each week will contain valuable insights and information.

Week 1:

Week one is made up of four steps that will focus on pretreatment instructions, as well as setting some personal goals, eating for healing inflammation, choosing the right supplements, and much more.

You will learn about the following:

1) Goals and the Motivation Behind Those Goals

As you go through this course, you will need the right mind-set to build a rock-solid foundation toward achieving your goals. Remember to slow down, dive deeper than the surface to find your answers, include close people in your life, and pray and meditate. Accept that as you reach your goals, you will have new ones.

To achieve your goals, you must have the motivation for each goal, so take the time to write down what your personal motivation is. The setting of your goals and motivation is not something to put off, and always remember that nothing worthwhile is easy. We are going to teach you to:

- Understand your goals
- Repeat your goals out loud
- Find your personal motivation for your goals
- Evaluate your goals
- Reward yourself

2) Cellular Healing and Eating Right

By the time you get to this lesson, you will have had your new stem cells injected. Now it is time to learn how to create a healing environment for those cells to grow and replicate the best they can. The cellular healing diet is a breakthrough eating plan that, potentially, is the answer you've been praying for. We are going to teach you:

- What to eat and what not to eat
- How to avoid overeating
- How much water you need to drink and when
- What to do when you are emotionally upset
- How to cook vegetables and eat raw ones
- How to make eating an enjoyable time
- How to read food labels!
- How to limit fats and sweets and prepare wholesome snacks
- How to lower the outside stress in your life

Be good to yourself. Your decision to improve the quality of your life through healthier food choices and meal planning is a very significant step toward better health. You are in control. By taking care of your body through good health habits and fitness, you will live a happier, better, and longer life!

3) Recipes

In this lesson, we will discuss many different food choices and offer recipes that are tasty and easy to make. Nutrition is an essential part of good health, but most people ignore good nutrition until a disease develops that forces them to look at the food they eat. I want to change the way you look at food and give you a better understanding of what good nutrition really means. We are going to teach you about the following:

- Smoothies and juice can offer your body the nutrients and fuel it needs
- The tricks and common-sense way to use green smoothies.
- Recipes for the slow cooker
- Why you need to drink bone broth
- How to cleanse your body in a way that is both safe and tasty

4) Reading Food Labels

In this lesson, you will learn how to decipher those labels and read between the lines. Understanding the claims and what they mean will give you the power to make better decisions on the food you buy for yourself and your family. We are going to teach you:

- How to really read food labels
- How corporate food companies stretch that truth to sell you
- What is a correct serving size?
- Why you need quality over quantity
- The truth about sweeteners

5) Supplements and Nutrients

In this lesson, we will talk about which supplements you should take and which ones you should not take. There are certain recommendations on which supplements to take after stem cells, so it keeps on enhancing the stem cells after therapy.

Week 2:

This lesson is an exciting one! We will be learning all about a tapping technique known as EFT, which is short for Emotional Freedom Technique. It was originally developed by Roger Callahan in the early 1980s. He was a psychologist at Stanford University at the time he developed the tapping technique. Since that time, many different forms and techniques have been used. It is estimated that over one million people have had life-transforming success with the various techniques.

The way it works is that Dr. Callahan believed that each negative thought has a corresponding spot or meridian point located somewhere on the body. By applying pressure in the correct series, while mentally focusing on those thoughts, it is possible to alter negative emotions. This is a technique used for pain relief, phobias, breaking bad habits, weight loss, and more.

We will also reinforce or help to establish morning and evening rituals that will benefit your overall health. I am going to help you establish the foundation for lifelong habits that you can adapt both in the morning and evening.

These are some of the things you will learn:

- How EFT tapping works
- Sample EFT phrases
- The first thing you should do when you wake up
- Why it is important to start your day positive
- Meditation exercises
- Other routines such as oil pulling, skin brushing, etc.
- Why you need good oral hygiene
- How to wind down your day
- How to exercise
- Creating a good sleep routine

Week 3:

This week will be about stretching and strengthening your core muscles. In these lessons, we will discuss the multiple benefits of stretching and exercises specifically to strengthen your core muscles. While it is great that you are doing any exercise at all, it is important to get the most benefit from your efforts. People are busier today with careers, family, and more. One of the main reasons people have for not exercising is time, or rather, the lack of it. Three to four times a week, only twenty minutes of time is all it takes!

Here is some of the information included:

- The most up-to-date health and fitness information from my own clinical experience
- Other experts' research on fitness
- Simple five-minute stretching routines
- Exercises specific to core strengthening
- Water exercises for those with weight issues

Week 4:

Eating is a necessity of life. Every single living thing on earth must eat. Food brings together family and friends as well as providing comfort. Yet it is also a part of the growing epidemic of obesity that is, in turn, a cause of heart disease and diabetes, taking people's lives years earlier than otherwise would happen.

In this lesson, we will talk about intermittent fasting, which has been scientifically proven, and is centered on WHEN to eat. Unlike a regular fast, you will not be missing thousands of calories in a day. Instead, you simply eat all your meals in a shorter amount of time.

In this lesson, we will also be discussing one of the most crucial functions of your body for any level of health. Elimination or bowel movements. How much waste product can the average body hold? The GI (gastrointestinal) tract, colon, and intestines are estimated to have a total combined capacity of sixty pounds!

This is some of the information you will learn:

- When and how to fast
- The science behind intermittent fasting
- Tips for successful fasting
- Short- and long-term fasting benefits
- How to remove constipation in three steps
- The link to colon cancer
- All about laxatives
- What you want to look for in your poo
- Colon and digestive health

Week 5:

Week five is about energy and the power of the mind. We will explore Qigong, a 6000-year-old exercise focused on the movement of energy. It helps with organs, heart, liver, and kidneys, and this exercise is helpful in strengthening the shoulder and knee joints.

Qi is energy, but more than that, it is relating.

Gong is the movement of energy.

Meditation is also an essential part of our enhancement program. Focused breathing and setting out a time to be mindful goes a long way toward propelling you into healing and rejuvenation. I will also be sharing an app I give to my patients for meditation.

You will learn how to do the following:

- Pay attention to the flow of energy
- Practice breathing and warming up
- Acknowledge your thoughts

- Create a meditative environment
- Be mindful of breath and body
- Stretch and breathe deeply
- Perform the eight brocades

Week 6:

The final week covers sleep, which is essential to good health. With a focus on how to sleep more deeply, we work with patients to make sure they get more, high-quality rest. We are also going to discuss an exciting new cartilage-rebuilder supplement. This is not simply taking glucosamine chondroitin, but an actual Chinese medicine to rid the body of arthritis.

This is what you will learn:

- There is not a single ailment, mental or physical, that is not made worse by the lack of sleep
- How each of the five stages of sleep plays a vital role in your health
- A process of retraining your brain and body to sleep in a natural pattern that is healthy
- How to set a new, healthy sleep pattern for yourself
- The importance of establishing a bedtime routine
- Sleep distractions and how to avoid them
- What foods to avoid before bed
- A new cartilage-rebuilder supplement to rid the body of arthritis

Healing and Hope through the Enhancement Program

After graduation from the enhancement program, patients often feel heightened healing and hope. We are not done yet though, as we continue to surround you with support. As the program ends, we book two follow-up appointments, at week six and at week twelve. This gives us the opportunity to check in with you and fine-tune any aspect you still need help with.

It goes hand in hand as part of the healing process, and I don't want you to underestimate the importance of having a post-stem cell therapy plan. The enhancement program includes a series of video lessons with a manual, so patients can maximize their knowledge of their health conditions.

Our Gift to You

Of course, in our office, this enhancement program is part of our stem cell therapy procedure for all our patients. We are offering our stem cell patients, a **complimentary, six-week, video enhancement program**. If you have had stem cell injections, we want to give you the very best chance possible to not only heal, but to allow those stem cells to regenerate to their full potential. This is a free gift to our patients.

However, the enhancement program is also available to anyone. For those people who may have received stem cell therapy *at another clinic,* we want to help you as well, and you are welcome to *purchase the enhancement program* through www.regenhealthmed.com by clicking "Start Here."

Whatever happens, know that there is hope, and you can find healing. By understanding and examining all aspects of your health, you can basically supercharge your stem cell therapy experience by boosting your personal health and wellness.

Give Your Health Every Advantage

As a doctor who looks at every patient from a whole health perspective, my best outcome is working one on one with each individual client on a long-term health plan. Having only so many hours in the day, and I am not able to physically discuss every single person's condition and circumstances.

When I realized that, I quickly decided to make information available to those who I am not able to see personally. That is what this book, my website and other resources are all about—the best health for everyone.

Stem cell therapy is so versatile, and as you can read from the success stories I have shared, patients have seen remarkable results. At the same time, stem cell therapy works more effectively on patients who take a different approach to their health. Once people realize how the systems of their body work in synchronicity, they can become healthier.

Seeing this pattern in my many years of helping people, over and over the same specific products were showing health advantages in conjunction with stem cell therapy. Based on this perspective, over time I simplified the process for my patients with a supplement that improved three key areas of health, directly related to what the stem cells were already doing.

My goal, is to improve my patient's whole health and wanted to find a way for their stem cells to work better. We're going to put new resources into their body. If those stem cells can't get to the place where their body needs it, then it's not going to be effective. And if their environment and their body is very inflammatory, they are not going to benefit to the peak their body is capable of. This is why the StemVantage supplement was formulated, to give your body the advantage it needs.

Maximizing Stem Cell Benefits

In order to set the stage biochemically within your body, for the stem cells to circulate through the blood and reach the target area, specific cellular enhancements can provide a health boost. By following research on key areas that enhance cellular function, and applying it to the patients I see every day, I was able to isolate a supplement that helps produce positive results.

What it comes down to, is preparing the body's systems to receive cells through good circulation and other health indicators. We need to have the cells ready to accept these healing properties. And that's the point of the ingredients in StemVantage. It is to achieve that goal of optimal health.

Improve Circulation

Since stem cells travel through the blood stream, circulation is a big part of the process. Every ingredient in this supplement is involved in improved circulation. From garlic to olive leaf, and Ginkgo, they all work in the body to help our circulation.

The effects of Ginkgo Biloba, especially to the brain through the carotid artery, has been seen to improve circulation systemically throughout the entire body as well in the brain. Seeing the need for a healthy circulation system, this was a benefit I wanted for all of my patients. They are getting that with this formula.

From there, I formulated the supplement to include things that will help the cell function; the normal, anti-oxidant activity, like vitamin D, some of the bioflavonoids, which allow the cells to not continue to be damaged. Working together, these ingredients are not necessarily mitigating inflammation, but just trying to stop the oxidative damage. In that way, the stem cells we have injected, will have a healthier environment to survive in.

Isolate Nutrients that Enhance Cellular Repair

Every aspect of StemVantage, was added after careful consideration and close study. Taking the most recent research and implementing it in our patient's health programs, the result was enhanced cellular repair.

A recent study saw that using olive leaf extract, which is the Oleuropin with Hematopoietic stem cells (HSCs), allows stem cells to stimulate their self-renewal and provides the first evidence of the potential differentiation effect of olive leaf compounds on stem cells. So the science shows that by adding this supplement with the stem cell therapy, it is causing the conversion of them into the proper tissue, which allows them to get to the right place, at the highest possible rate. What that means is, it helps the stem cell convert to what it's supposed to convert to.

Increase Cellular Longevity

Another prominent study shows that you can modulate the cell death in modulate cytokines at the same time you're calming down inflammation once it's there. You are keeping the cells active longer, which is the perfect situation for stem cell therapy to be successful. In this particular case, they were studying it for leukemia, but again, the point of it was it had an effect on the stem cell reaction.

Therefore, because you're preventing cell death with this, which is tremendous, you're helping the stem cells live longer because that's what is directly affecting their life span. Many of these effects can be contributed to production of cytokines. You're going from the cellular level back out not from pushing it down with an artificial drug and, it's allowing the body to work as it's supposed to in its optimal condition. This allows the stem cells the greatest chance to survive and convert.

One Supplement – Three Positive Effects

We know the stem cell therapy works for a broad range of patients. Now we use StemVantage to encourage an optimal environment. We are trying to give each stem cell injected the greatest chance of getting to where they are supposed to go, and living long enough to reach its destination.

Why am I even suggesting that you should use a supportive supplement? Isn't just the stem cell therapy alone enough? Stem cells are enough, but I want to give you the best advantage.

StemVantage is not a substitute for getting stem cells, but it is used after stem cell therapy to provide the best advantage through:

- Circulation to where they are needed in the body
- Surviving in a non-hostile body
- Regenerating in the required way

We need to give those new stem cells the greatest chance of helping the patient. Don't you agree? Think of this supplement as a way to help them find their path for the best possible outcome.

Then from that point, we need to improve their circulation, get new blood to flow, then bring the nutrients that allows them to start the process of conversion. You want them to live as long as they can and keep those cells alive, so they don't die in the process of converting.

And then to allow the new cell to live, you want to create the greatest possible environment for that cell to survive, which means you want to have good, strong antioxidant support, and good circulation to allow nutrients to come in.

This product is better than any of the stem cell supplements out there, because it was created to give stem cells the greatest chance to work. It was formulated specifically for treating the overall health in a mutually beneficial way.

Part of a Whole Health Approach

This supplement is part of a whole health approach, based on how stem cells work in order to give them the greatest chance of survival and conversion.

We have tested this supplement over and over with people, and we have also seen results on patients who used different products. So rather than your body having to deal with absorbing or not absorbing or contradicting anything else; you will receive exactly what you need in the right amounts, rather than picking out something close and kind of making it work.

This supplement works for you based on the way stem cells work to regenerate and improve overall health. Through the creation of this supplement, I am helping patients by positivity changing the environment where the stem cells can actually do their work.

Go to
www.NutriHealthLabs.com
to get StemVantage.

And use the discount code:
"save30"
to get $30 off your 1st purchase.

https://www.ncbi.nlm.nih.gov/pmc/articles/PMC3163160/

https://www.ncbi.nlm.nih.gov/pubmed/21928670

https://www.ncbi.nlm.nih.gov/pmc/articles/PMC2775070/

INDEX

Dr. Raj Banerjee D.C.

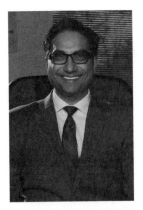

Dr. Raj Banerjee is a leading expert on health and wellness. He resides in St. Louis, Missouri where he is the clinic director of Regenerative Health Medicine of St. Louis, LLC. He specializes in customizing natural treatment programs targeting an array of health issues.

Dr. Banerjee leverages over 18+ years of extensive clinical experience in his practice, seeing over 8,000 patients, possessing a particular interest in nonsurgical and minimally invasive procedures. He incorporates the latest emerging techniques into his repertoire of services, so patients with chronic health conditions can get started on their path to total health and healing.

He is compassionate about whole body health and helping people no one else can treat. Using a personalized approach to nutrition, health and lifestyle, he has empowered people to reclaim their health and quality of life. Now with Regenerative Medicine, he can do even more to end the suffering of people with chronic conditions. When a body is healthy at a cellular level, the body can heal itself.

For more information on becoming a patient
or starting the Stem Cell Enhancement Program
please visit:

www.RegenHealthMed.com/StartHere

or Call:
314-282-3990

For more information on the newest stem
cell supplement called StemVantage please visit:

www.NutriHealthLabs.com

Use discount code

"save30"

to save $30 on your first
purchase of StemVantage.

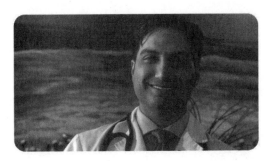

The latest state-of-the-art healing procedure...
REGENERATIVE STEM CELL THERAPY

The Regenerative Health Medicine of St. Louis team, is a collaboration of MDs, orthopedic surgeons and other health professionals, working together to provide wellness options for people struggling with autoimmune, chronic pain and other issues.

Learn what years of experiences has taught us:

- How Stem Cell therapy is helping people with knee and joint pain find relief after only one treatment!

- How this remarkable cutting edge healing technology that can actually repair damaged tissue in the body through a painless and safe stem cell injection.

- According to Regenerative Health Medicine of St. Louis's chief medical officer, "Patients can experience a significant decrease in pain and improved range of motion within weeks of just one treatment." When the body heals, the pain naturally goes away.

- Discover how stem cell injections work... (This is really fascinating stuff!) We'll explain how they pinpoint the impaired areas, remove the swelling with powerful anti-inflammatory properties and heal them by regenerating new cells and tissue.

- Why this innovative therapy is helpful for degenerative arthritis, degenerative cartilage and ligaments, bone spurs, degenerative joint disease bursitis and tendinitis.

If you or someone you know, suffers from joint pain, or any one of these aliments this could be a life-changing therapy

Dr. Raj Banerjee

For more information on becoming a patient or starting
the Stem Cell Enhancement Program please visit:
www.RegenHealthMed.com/StartHere

For more information on the newest stem cell supplement
called StemVantage please visit: www.NutriHealthLabs.com

Use discount code "save30" to save $30 on
your first purchase of StemVantage.